Psychotherapy and Psychosomatics

Founded 1953 as 'Acta Psychotherapeutica et Psychosomatica'
by E.A.D.E. Carp and B. Stokvis, continued by
Th. Spoerri (1964–1974) and P.E. Sifneos (1974–1991)

KARGER

Printed in Switzerland
on acid-free paper by
Thür AG Offsetdruck, Pratteln

Appears 6-weekly:
2 volumes per year (8 issues)

Psychotherapy and Psychosomatics

Submission: Only original papers written in English are considered and should be sent to:

Giovanni A. Fava
Dipartimento di Psicologìa
Università di Bologna
Viale Berti Pichat 5
I- 40127 Bologna (Italia)

Manuscripts should be submitted in triplicate (with three sets of illustrations of which one is an original), typewritten double-spaced on one side of the paper, with a wide margin.

Conditions: All manuscripts are subject to editorial review. Manuscripts are received with the explicit understanding that they are not under simultaneous consideration by any other publication. Submission of an article for publication implies the transfer of the copyright from the author to the publisher upon acceptance. Accepted papers become the permanent property of 'Psychotherapy and Psychosomatics' and may not be reproduced by any means, in whole or in part, without the written consent of the publisher. It is the author's responsibility to obtain permission to reproduce illustrations, tables, etc. from other publications.

Arrangement

Title page: The first page of each paper should indicate the title (main title underlined), the authors' names, and the institute where the work was conducted. A short title for use as running head as well as the full address of the author to whom correspondence should be sent are also required.

Full address: The exact postal address complete with postal code must be given at the bottom of the title page. Please supply also Phone and Fax numbers.

Key words: For indexing purposes, a list of 4–10 key words in English is essential.

Abstract: Each paper needs an abstract of up to 10 lines.

Small type: Paragraphs which can or must be set in smaller type (case histories, test methods, etc.) should be indicated with a 'p' (petit) in the margin on the left-hand side.

Footnotes: Avoid footnotes. When essential, they are numbered consecutively and typed at the foot of the appropriate page.

Tables and illustrations: Tables and illustrations (both numbered in Arabic numerals) should be prepared on separate sheets. Tables require a heading and figures a legend, also prepared on a separate sheet. For the reproduction of illustrations, only good drawings and original photographs can be accepted; negatives or photocopies cannot be used. When possible, group several illustrations on one block for reproduction (max. size 144 × 196 mm) or provide crop marks. On the back of each illustration, indicate its number, the author's name, and 'top'. Color illustrations are reproduced at the author's expense.

References: In the text identify references by Arabic numerals [in square brackets]. Material submitted for publication but not yet accepted should be noted as 'unpublished data' and not be included in the reference list. The list of references should include only those publications which are cited in the text. Do not alphabetize; number references in the order in which they are first mentioned in the text. The surnames of the authors followed by initials should be given. There should be no punctuation other than a comma to separate the authors. Cite all authors, 'et al' is not sufficient. Abbreviate journal names according to the Index Medicus system. (Also see International Committee of Medical Journal Editors: Uniform requirements for manuscripts submitted to biomedical journals. Br Med J 1988;296:401–405.)

Examples

(a) Papers published in periodicals: Kauffman HF, van der Heide S, Beaumont F, Blok H, de Vries K: Class-specific antibody determination against *Aspergillus fumigatus* by means of the enzyme-linked immunosorbent assay. III. Comparative study: IgG, IgA, IgM ELISA titers, precipitating antibodies and IgE binding after fractionation of the antigen. Int Arch Allergy Appl Immunol 1986;80:300–306.

(b) Monographs: Matthews DE, Farewell VT: Using and Understanding Medical Statistics. Basel, Karger, 1985.

(c) Edited books: Hardy WD Jr, Essex M: FeLV-induced feline acquired immune deficiency syndrome: A model for human AIDS; in Klein E (ed): Acquired Immunodeficiency Syndrome. Prog Allergy. Basel, Karger, 1986, vol 37, pp 353–376.

Further details: Authors may consult our leaflet 'Rules for the Preparation of Manuscripts', available on request from the Publisher, S. Karger AG, P.O. Box, CH-4009 Basel (Switzerland).

Page charges: There is no page charge for papers of 7 or fewer printed pages (including tables, illustrations and references). Each additional complete or partial page is charged to the author at SFr. 225.– / US $ 150.00. The allotted size of a paper is equal to approx. 16 manuscript pages (including tables, illustrations and references).

Galley proofs: Unless indicated otherwise, galley proofs are sent to the first-named author and should be returned with the least possible delay. Alterations made in galley proofs, other than the correction of printer's errors, are charged to the author. No page proofs are supplied.

Reprints: Order forms and a price list are sent with the galley proofs. Orders submitted after the issue is printed are subject to considerably higher prices. Allow five weeks from date of publication for delivery of reprints.

KARGER

General Information

Psychotherapy and Psychosomatics

Publication data: 'Psychotherapy and Psychosomatics' is published 8 times annually. Volumes 57–58 with 4 issues each appear in 1992.

Subscription rates: Subscriptions run for a full calendar year. Prices are given per volume, surface postage included.

Personal subscription:
SFr. 179.20, US$ 119.70.
(Must be in the name of, billed to, and paid by an individual. Order must be marked 'personal subscription'.)

Institutional subscription:
(Regular rate.) SFr. 256.–, US$ 171.00.

Members of the American Psychological Association; International Federation for Medical Psychotherapy:
SFr. 153.60, US$ 102.60.

Airmail postage: SFr. 25.–, US$ 20.00.
(Extra per volume.)

Microform subscription:
SFr. 128.–, US$ 85.50.
(Available exclusively to subscribers of the paper edition.)

Single issues and back volumes: Information on availability and prices can be obtained through the Publisher.

Advertising: Correspondence and rate requests should be addressed to the Publisher.

Subscription orders: Orders can be placed at agencies, bookstores, directly with the Publisher S. Karger AG, P.O. Box, CH – 4009 Basel (Switzerland) or with any of the following distributors:

Deutschland:
S. Karger GmbH, Lörracher Strasse 16A
Postfach, D-W–7800 Freiburg

France: Librairie Luginbühl
36, bd de Latour-Maubourg,
F – 75007 Paris

Great Britain, Ireland:
S. Karger Publishers
11 Ravenscroft Road
Beckenham, Kent BR3 4TP

USA: S. Karger Publishers, Inc.
26 West Avon Road, P.O. Box 529
Farmington, CT 06085

India, Bangladesh, Sri Lanka:
S. Karger India Subscription Agency
B – 5/132 Safdarjung Enclave
New Delhi-110029

Japan: Katakura Libri, Inc.
36-9 Hongo 3-chome, Bunkyo-ku
Tokyo 113

Change of address: Both old and new address should be stated and sent to the subscription source.

Bibliographic indices: This journal is regularly listed in bibliographic services, including *Current Contents®*.

Book Reviews: Books are accepted for review by special agreement.

Unique references for dealing with psychosomatic disorders

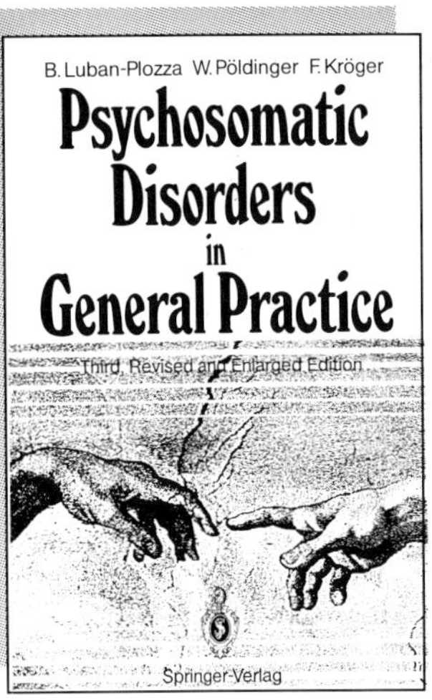

B. Luban-Plozza,
Locarno;
W. Pöldinger,
University of Basel,
F. Kröger,
RWTH Aachen

Psychosomatic Disorders in General Practice

Translated and revised from the German by G. Blythe

Foreword by M. Balint

3rd, rev. and enlarged ed. 1992. XII, 255 pp. 18 figs. 18 tabs. Softcover DM 68,– ISBN 3-540-54556-5

The practice-oriented approach of this book brought its previous editions wide acclaim. It has now been thoroughly revised and expanded in this third edition.

The authors present the basic knowledge of psychosomatics that both specialists and nonspecialists require, and then show how this knowledge is applied in practice by putting the theoretical concepts underlying psychosomatics into a practical context with descriptions of psychosomatic illnesses. The various therapeutic approaches to the patient, ranging from discussions between patient and physician to Balint group work and family therapy, are all discussed.

This new edition is suitable for use as a basic introduction, giving practical guidance on basic psychosomatic care of patients both in the practice and in the clinic.

J. W. Paulley, H. E. Pelser

Psychological Managements for Psychosomatic Disorders

Foreword by J. J. Groen

1989. XVI, 335 pp. 15 figs. Softcover DM 98,–
ISBN 3-540-19298-0

"... The authors' main aim is to set out the precise psychological management appropriate to each disorder.... The theory of illness presented here is determinism at its finest, with typical patients, in psychological terms, destined to have a particular physical disorder as soon as they meet the appropriate emotional stresses...

We are all used to such determinism in our models of the natural history of external risk and illness outcome, but it is discomforting to see this approach applied so vigorously to the human mind as a risk factor for physical disease. Paulley and Pelser offer a detailed and intelligent explanation for our discomfort in their final chapter, a splendid blast from the past and a robust attack on "the retreat from patients", fashions in medical training, ultraspecialisation, and holistic medicine. Great stuff.

Why not try this experiment? Ask your patients with asthma, multiple sclerosis, or rheumatoid arthritis whether they think that emotional stress helped to make them ill. Some will surprise you with a detailed and highly personal psychosomatic explanation, previously unrevealed. If you want to pursue the matter, read this book, which is based on a wealth of conviction and experience.
Two poignant questions remain: how does one prove and quantify a psychosomatic aetiology, and how rigorous is the evidence offered here?"

The Lancet

Prices are subject to change without notice

Psychotrauma

2nd European Conference
on Traumatic Stress,
Noordwijkerhout,
The Netherlands,
September 23–27, 1990

Editors
Wolter S. De Loos,
Leiden
Wybrand Op den Velde,
Amsterdam

5 figures and 17 tables, 1992

KARGER

S. Karger
Medical and Scientific Publishers
Basel · Freiburg · Paris · London
New York · New Delhi · Bangkok
Singapore · Tokyo · Sydney

Drug Dosage
The authors and the publisher have exerted every effort to ensure that drug selection and dosage set forth in this text are in accord with current recommendations and practice at the time of publication. However, in view of ongoing research, changes in government regulations, and the constant flow of information relating to drug therapy and drug reactions, the reader is urged to check the package insert for each drug for any change in indications and dosage and for added warnings and precautions. This is particularly important when the recommended agent is a new and/or infrequently employed drug.

P.O. Box, CH–4009 Basel (Switzerland)
Printed in Switzerland on acid-free paper by
Thür AG Offsetdruck, Pratteln
ISBN 3–8055–5662–4

Contents

2nd Europ Conf on Traumatic Stress
Psychother Psychosom 1992;57:141–142

Guest Editors
Wolter S. De Loos
Wybrand Op den Velde
Leiden/Amsterdam

Foreword

Psychologists and psychiatrists have long ignored the fact that shocking and severely distressing events can have a lasting impact. It was only in 1980 that a properly defined diagnostic category, describing the sequelae of traumatic experiences, was proposed and found general acceptance. The introduction of this category of posttraumatic stress disorders (PTSD) in DSM-III marks the revival of interest in psychological trauma as a cause of psychopathology. Only 10 years later 'classical' PTSD, as opposed to other posttraumatic syndromes, is generally recognized as a diagnostic category.

The First European Conference on Traumatic Stress was held in Lincoln, UK, in 1988 and was followed in 1990 by the second conference under this title, held in Noordwijkerhout, The Netherlands. The aim of the organizers was to bring together European health care professionals working with victims of psychological violence. Even if judged only by the increase in the number of participants, from 115 in 1988 to 500 two years later, the conference was obviously considered to fulfill a need. And there are further pointers signifying an increase of interest in the subject, at least in Western societies. In the last decade local and national study groups and an increasing number of postacademic courses on psychotrauma have emerged. The interest in victimology, incest, child battering, war victims, refugees, rehabilitation after torture, occupational trauma, traffic and transport accidents, and other disasters has increased noticeably. And, last but not least, in 1985 the Society for Traumatic Stress Studies was founded in the USA, which in 1991 adopted the prefix 'International' and publishes the *Journal of Traumatic Stress.*

The Second European Conference on Traumatic Stress also met an early but distinct desire for communication with Eastern European couuntries, after their liberation from oppressive regimes. The organizing committee was able to support a considerable number of delegates from these countries enabling them to attend the conference and to develop mutually beneficial contacts.

Out of a total of 180 contributions presented at the Second European Conference on Traumatic Stress only a limited number will be published. Some contribuitons will appear in *Anxiety Research: An International Journal* [4: 183–254], edited by HM van der Ploeg. A number of studies on the impact of psychotraumatic events on members of the police force will be published as: *Police Symposium,* edited by BPR Gersons, IVE Carlier, GCK Vlek, in the series: Politie en Trauma (Police and Trauma), ed. GCK Vlek. Den Haag, Ministerie van Binnenlandse Zaken, Directie Politie, 1992.

In this issue of *Psychotherapy and Psychosomatics* a selection of articles based on contributions to the Second European Conference on Traumatic Stress is presented, which demonstrate the diversity in the field of psychotraumatology. Three contributions deal with respectively traumatization as a result of incest during childhood (Albach and Everaerd), intrafamilial violence (Black et al.), and shipwreck (Yule). Members of the armed forces are the subject of an article on Swedish members of the United Nations peace keeping forces, whose work is of a very complicated nature and gives rise to many conflicts (Lundin and Otto). A number of contributions deal with survivors of the Second World War, suffering from lasting chronic posttraumatic symptoms. One article examines the relation between the specific features of posttraumatic stress disorders and certain other psychological symptoms (Hovens et al.); another one concerning a cohort of resistance veterans in their fifth decade after the war describes the difficult psychosomatic problem of cardiovascular risk in relation to posttraumatic stress disorder (Falger et al.); the third describes a psychopharmacological study in this cohort, which appears to be very resistant to therapy (De Boer et al.). Somatic reenactment in the treatment of posttraumatic stress disorder (Lindy et al.) is another aspect that hitherto has not attracted much attention. And finally, an ethological study (Wiepkema and Schouten) on a symptom observed in maltreated domestic animals illustrates the relevance of comparative biology to the understanding of possible parallels with posttraumatic states in human childhood. Apparently, this symptom is related to the psychobiology of opioids which most probably play an important role in the generation of posttraumatic symptoms.

The scientific and practical field of psychotraumatology developed very rapidly during the last decade. The Conference made it clear that psychotraumatology overlaps with many scientific disciplines. Psychotrauma is now recognized to be a major cause of psychosocial dysfunctioning. Apart from the propensity to cause the distressing symptoms of 'classical' PTSD, psychological trauma may have a profound impact on the life style and relations of the victims and on their personal systems of beliefs.

Finally, it is a pleasure to acknowledge the germane and obliging assistance of the editorial advisors in the process of reviewing the manuscripts. We also thank Dr. H.E. Pelser for his aid to the writing of this foreword.

2nd Europ Conf on Traumatic Stress
Psychother Psychosom 1992;57:143–151

Francine Albach
Walter Everaerd

Department of Clinical Psychology, Faculty of Psychology, University of Amsterdam, The Netherlands

Posttraumatic Stress Symptoms in Victims of Childhood Incest

Key Words
Incest
Trauma
Posttraumatic stress disorder

Abstract
The relationship between posttraumatic stress disorder (PTSD) and the experience of severe childhood incest was investigated in a comparison of 97 adult female victims of incest and 65 matched controls. It appeared that 62% of the incest victims and none of the controls met the DSM-III-R criteria for PTSD. The best predictor for the development of PTSD appeared to be the subjective reaction at the time of the event, consisting of anxiety, freezing and dissociation. The incest victims also displayed other psychiatric symptoms, such as self-mutilation and conversions. Although the relation incest-PTSD is quite obvious, the diagnosis may easily be missed because the symptoms may be masked by other psychiatric phenomena.

Introduction

We know from literature that victims of incest may suffer from many psychiatric symptoms [1–3]. They may display self-destructive behavior [4, 5], substance abuse [4], dissociative phenomena [6], and hysterical symptoms such as a conversion disorder [7] and sexually provocative behaviour [8]. Victims of childhood traumas could be given different diagnoses such as borderline personality, conduct disorder, phobic disorder, dissociative disorder, panic disorder, posttraumatic stress disorder (PTSD) and multiple personality disorder [9]. According to Terr [9], there is no diagnosis which fully describes the sequelae of childhood abuse or incest. Nevertheless, it seems possible to argue that victims of incest meet criteria for the diagnosis of PTSD.

If psychiatry officially recognised (some of) the symptoms as belonging to PTSD, this would mean that experiences of incest would be finally acknowledged as just as important

Dr. F. Albach
Marnixstraat 291
NL–1015 WL Amsterdam (The Netherlands)

0033–3190/92/
0574–0143$2.75/0

as acts of violence or atrocities in war. It would also mean that victims of incest could benefit from existing knowledge about the therapy of PTSD.

For a long time, this has been prevented by the fact that psychiatrists tended to disbelieve reports about incest and considered these stories to be lies [10]. Today the situation is different, although it will always be problematic to be a hundred percent sure about what happened, incest being a crime where in most cases no witnesses are present and where the perpetrator will deny his acts. When a victim tells about her experiences, she is believed [7] and is often referred to a special incest group. There is however no guarantee that her symptoms will also be recognised and that her PTSD will be treated. One of the authors observed that even in therapy groups for incest victims no attention was being paid to symptoms of PTSD such as flashbacks, nightmares or startle responses. In these groups the fact that these women all had experienced incestuous abuse was common knowledge. But the possibility that they might also suffer from PTSD symptoms was not recognised, although on the basis of our knowledge of other traumatized individuals [11] and on the basis of some studies about victims of incest [12, 13] it could be expected that incest would lead to posttraumatic symptoms.

Besides PTSD, victims of incest may display various other symptoms and therefore there is the problem of comorbidity: the presence of these other symptoms may mask their PTSD. This is a general problem with traumatized individuals who suffer from PTSD (like war veterans, who may be considered as alcoholics [14]).

The etiological significance of the incest for the development of the later PTSD is also problematic. When is it most likely that a victim of incest will develop PTSD? Which are the best predictors for the development of PTSD? We know from the literature that the severer kinds of incest are the types of abuse which happen more than once or which go on for years. Those which start at an early age and which have to be kept secret; where the father is the perpetrator; in which coitus takes place or where the child has to masturbate the man; and in which force and/or violence is used [15, 16]. The impact of these events is made worse by the characteristics of the incestuous families. Often incest is accompanied by role reversal (the child is held responsible for the emotional wellbeing of the parent (emotional role reversal), or has to keep house (functional role reversal) [17]. Also, the subjective reaction to the event may play an important role. Both a reaction of anxiety and distress [18] and of the defense against this anxiety, i.e. a reaction of 'freezing' [19] and dissociation [20] are supposed to add to the later development of PTSD. Therefore, it may be assumed that the subjective reaction to the event and the duration, age of onset, secrecy, relationship with the perpetrator, severity of the sexual acts or of the force which was used are all useful predictors for the eventual development of PTSD.

The following study was done because we think that it is important both to discover whether victims of incest do suffer from PTSD (which may be masked by other psychiatric symptoms) and to know which characteristics of the incest are the best predictors for the development of PTSD. In this study, two groups were interviewed: a group which had experienced (the most severe kinds of) incest and a control group which was matched to the incest group for demographic characteristics.

The following problems were addressed: (1) Do incest victims display more PTSD symptoms than a comparable group of women who did not experience incest as a child? (2) Which characteristics of the incest situation are the best predictors for the later development of PTSD symptoms? (3) Is there a comorbidity with other psychiatric symptoms?

Method

Subjects

The study was carried out with two groups, a group of victims of incest and a control group without any experiences of incest. The respondents were recruited by the so-called 'snowball method'; initial respondents volunteering to cooperate were asked to put us into touch with others. When the control group respondent appeared to be a victim of incest during the interview, this interview was removed afterwards from the study and was not included in the analysis. In this way, a group of 97 female incest victims between the age of 18 and 55 and a matched control group of 65 women was obtained. Through the procedure of the snowball method we hoped to find women who had experienced the severest kinds of incest, because in this group most psychiatric symptoms could be expected.

Only females were studied, because from the literature it is known that the victims of incest are mainly girls [21]. Only adults were studied, as the aim of the research was to study the long-term PTSD. Those variables with which both groups were matched included sex, age, educational level and social background of the parents of the person. Other variables, such as being married or having children, were excluded from the matching procedure. Given that one of the consequences of incest is the fear and avoidance of men, it can be expected that fewer incest victims will be married and have children than 'normal' women. The incest and the control group appeared to be similar in the demographic characteristics of sex, age, level of education and social background of their parents. In order to test for significant differences, t tests were run on the above variables and no significant differences were found except for the variables of marriage and having children: the incest victims were not as often married and had fewer children than the control respondents. When analyzing the data, it appeared that three interviews from the incest group were useless: the interviews had not been recorded on tape. Two further interviews had to be removed from the control group, one because the respondent appeared to be the victim of incest and the other because she could not report any negative life event as a child. Inclusion of control subjects was decided on the basis of their response to the question about whether they had experienced a negative event as a child.

Instrument and Procedure

The instrument had the form of a prestructured in-depth interview which could be scored according to a yes-or-no format afterwards. The response categories of some variables were continuous (indicated in the text as c), but most of them were dichotomous (indicated as d). There was one open question in which a content analysis was done (indicated as o). Apart from the demographic variables, the following variables were studied: characteristics of the event, family characteristics, subjective reaction to the event and psychiatric symptoms.

Characteristics of the Event

Incest. Questions were asked about age of onset (c), age of last abuse (c) and duration (c). Kind of perpetrator (father (d), stepfather (d), uncle (d), grandfather (d), other family members or lodger (d)). Kind of sexual acts (harassment (d), masturbation of the perpetrator (d), attempt at penetration (d), penetration (d), fellatio (d) and anal penetration (d)). The three categories of masturbation of the perpetrator, fellatio and penetration were added in order to form a combined category (d) of severe sexual acts. In addition questions were asked about the type of force which was used (he just did it/I obeyed (d), he used constraint (d), he used violence (d)). The last two categories were added in order to form a combined category of physical force (c).

Negative Life Events. In the control group an open question was asked as to whether the subject had experienced a negative event as a child and a description of the event was request (O).

Subjective Reaction to the Event. On the basis of the literature about the subjective experience of traumatic events, three kinds of reactions were distinguished: anxiety [18], freezing [19] and dissociation [20]. Respondents were therefore asked whether at the time of the event they had experienced anxiety (d), freezing (keeping stiff during the event) (d), or dissociation (feeling as if one wasn't there, as if it wasn't real, etc.) (d). On the basis of these three categories, an analysis with a combination of these three variables was formed, which was called the traumatic reaction (c).

Family Characteristics

On the basis of the literature about role reversal [17] respondents were also asked about functional role reversal (the child had the main responsibility for the household). As taking care of the household may be supposed to be a greater burden for a younger than for an older child, a difference was made between functional role reversal before the age of 13 and before the age of 18 (functional role reversal <13 (d) and functional role reversal <18 (d)). Also questions were asked about the emotional role reversal by the father (d) and by the mother (d) (the child was held responsible for the emotional wellbeing of the parent).

Posttraumatic Stress Symptoms

In both groups questions were asked about posttraumatic stress symptoms. These were defined according to the DSM-III-R description [22]. Existing PTSD questionnaires (like the Mississippi scale for combat-related posttraumatic stress disorder [23] did not prove very useful, because they are meant for war veterans and because they do not concern traumatic events in childhood. The following posttraumatic symptoms were studied: (1) Symptoms of reexperiencing the event: intrusive recollections (d), distressing dreams (d), sudden acting or feeling as if the event is reoccurring (d) and intense distress at exposure to events that symbolize the traumatic event (d). (2) Symptoms of avoidance of the event: efforts to avoid feelings (d) or situation (d) associated with the event, psychogenic amnesia (d), feeling of detachment from others (d) and a restricted range of affect (d). (3) Symptoms of increased arousal: difficulty staying or falling asleep (d), irritability (d) or outbursts of anger (d), hypervigilance (d), exaggerated startle response (d) and physiological reactivity to events that resemble the traumatic event (d). Combined scores on PTSD (c) were computed according to the DSM-III-R, where the minimal score for Reliving symptoms is 1, for Avoidance symptoms 3 and for symptoms of Increased Arousal 2. Total PTSD scores (c) consist of a combination of the minimum scores on these three groups of symptoms. The total PTSD score served as an indication for a lifetime diagnosis of PTSD, which means that the respondents had suffered from these symptoms once in their lives (and were not necessarily still suffering from them at the time the interview took place). This is important, for in the different phases of their lives patients may display different symptoms. During a period in which they are denying the traumatic events more denial symptoms could be anticipated and 'reliving' symptoms could seem to be absent.

Other Psychiatric Symptoms

In additon a questionnaire was administered about the following psychiatric symptoms: Self-destructive behavior (anorexia (d), bulimia (d), alcohol abuse (d), self-mutilation (d) and suicide attempts (d)). Dissociative behavior: amnesia relating to recent events (d), such as amnesia of the following: things which one has done or written, journeys which one has made, places which one has visited and thoughts which one has had. Hysterical symptoms: fainting (d), temporary paralysis of limbs (d), hysterical seizures (d), sexually provocative behavior (d) and undiagnosable chronic pelvic pain (d).

Data Collection

The incest group was interviewed first and the controls were selected afterwards on the basis of the demographic characteristics of the incest group. The interviews were carried out by 6 female clinical psychologists during a period of 3 years. The interview took place at the homes of the respondents. They were asked to give informed consent. Respondents were requested to conduct the interview in private in the absence of spouse and children. They were also advised to organize some form of supportive help (by therapists or friends) after the interview, in case of emotional breakdown. All interviews were audiotaped and were then typed out.

Data Analysis

On the answers to the questions about the 'ordinary negative events' a content analysis was done on the basis of the different categories and an interscorer reliability was computed which appeared to be good ($r = 0.86$). T tests were done in order to find out whether the differences in role reversal and PTSD between the incest and the control group were significant and a stepwise regression analysis was carried out in order to compute the contribution of the different characteristics of the incest situation.

Results

Characteristics of Incest and Other Negative Life Events

Incest Experiences. The characteristics of the incest situation in most subjects of this group appeared to meet criteria for the severest kinds of incest: 69% started before the age of 10, 90% lasted 1 year or more, in 64% the child had to keep it a secret, in 67% the father was found to be the perpetrator, in 69% coitus took place, in 81% the child had to mastur-

Table 1. PTSD in incest and control group

	Incest group, % (n = 97)	Control group, % (n = 65)
Reexperience symptoms (score > 1 item)	93	1*
Avoidance symptoms (score > 3 items)	64	0*
Increased arousal (score > 2 items)	97	4*
Total PTSD (score A + B + C)	62	0*

* Differences between the incest and the control group significant at $p < 0.0001$.

bate the man, and in 42% violence was used. Such kinds of incest are more similar to the experiences as reported in the study by Frenken [26] than to the representative samples presented by Drayer [16].

'Ordinary Negative Life Events'. The experiences of the control group appeared to be quite diverse, ranging from experiences of betrayal by the parents (for instance: mother secretly read the child's diary) or others (child was teased at school), witnessing of punishments in the family (for instance: mother beats brother), parental quarrels, the witnessing of accidents (for instance: the child saw brother unconscious in hospital), to serious illness, accidents, serious illness of parents or the family members and (noviolent) death of parents or other family members.

Subjective Reaction to Incest. 85% of the incest victims indicated that they had been anxious during the abuse, 87% reported that they had had a reaction of 'freezing' during the abuse and 76% reported that they had reacted with dissociation. As all these reactions appeared to be highly correlated, a new variable was formed out of a combination of these three reactions, which was called the traumatic reaction. 60% of all incest victims had a score of at least one on this new variable.

Family Characteristics

Incest sometimes coincided with other negative family characteristics. Functional role reversal before and after the age on 13 was reported by 12 and 31% of the respondents, respectively. 20% indicated that there had been emotional role reversal between the subject and the father and 38% indicated this role reversal between the subject and her mother. The incidence of role reversal with the father in the group in which the father had been the perpetrator of the incest was 59%. In the control group, functional role reversal before and after the age of 13 was reported by 1 and 3% of the respondents, respectively. Emotional role reversal with the father was reported by 5% and with the mother by 23% of the respondents. T tests showed that the differences between all these kinds of role reversal between the incest and the control group were significant at a $p < 0.05$.

Table 2. Comorbidity of PTSD in incest victims

	Incest victims, % (PTSD score > 6; n = 61)
Self-destructive behavior	
Anorexia	38
Bulimia	28
Alcohol abuse	39
Self-mutilation	25
Suicide attempts	38
Dissociative phenomena	
Amnesia of recent events	31
Hysterical symptoms	
Fainting	5
(Temporary) paralysis of limbs	13
Hysterical seizures	30
Sexually provocative behavior	51
Chronic pelvic pain	23

Percentages are calculated on the cases that met the criteria of PTSD.

Posttraumatic Stress Symptoms

From table 1 we see that 93% of the incest group and 1% of the control group scored on the Reliving symptoms. 64% of the incest group and 2% of the controls scored on the Avoidance symptoms, and 97 versus 4% scored on symptoms of Increased Arousal. When the total PTSD score was computed (consisting of the combination of the three symptom clusters of PTSD) none of the controls and 62% of the incest group appeared to meet the criterium of PTSD, defined according to the DSM-III-R. When tested, all differences between the two groups (on the total PTSD score and on the three kinds of subscores) appeared to be significant at $p < 0.0001$.

PTSD Symptoms and Other Psychiatric Symptoms

The respondents from the incest group who met the criteria for PTSD were scored for additional psychiatric symptoms. It appeared that PTSD in incest victims may be accompanied by self-destructive behavior, dissociative phenomena and hysterical symptoms (table 2).

Contribution of Specific Characteristics of the Incest Situation

From a stepwise regression analysis it appeared that 3 variables explained the variance of the score of PTSD symptoms. In this analysis the following variables were included: duration, age of onset, secrecy, father or stepfather as perpetrator, intimacy of sexual acts, severity of the force which was used, role reversal with the father, role reversal with the mother and the subjective traumatic reaction reported to have taken place during the event. The subjective reaction to the traumatic event was the first variable to be entered and this variable explained 30% of the variance. The variables of the second step and of the third step did not add much to the amount of explained variance (only 0.02 and 0.01 respectively). The variable of the second step appeared to consist of the severity of the sexual acts which the child had to comply with (manual and oral masturbation and vaginal penetration). The variable of the third step was the duration of the abuse.

Discussion

In this study, a group of women was interviewed which appeared to have been the victim of severer kinds of long-lasting sexual childhood abuse, which had consisted of very intimate kinds of sexual acts, and in which often (67%) the father had been the perpetrator. Compared to a representative sample of Dutch incest victims [16], the women in this group were extremely traumatized. On the basis of these experiences 62% had developed PTSD symptoms. In contrast, no woman from the matched control group met the criteria for PTSD. The negative life events which this group had experienced did not induce either intrusive reexperiences or any of the other PTSD symptoms. Therefore, it may be concluded that incest may lead to PTSD symptoms.

Similar results were found in other studies [4, 16]. In most of these studies, however, no attention was paid to the official PTSD symptoms (such as flashbacks, amnesia of the traumatic events etc.) and the authors did not try to establish whether the person suffered from PTSD as defined in DSM-III-R. Despite these differences, when predicting which individual victim of incest has the greatest chance of developing later symptoms, however, it is interesting to compare our results with theirs.

In this study the fact was again confirmed that the subjective reaction to the events is the best predictor for the development of later psychiatric problems [16]. In contrast to other studies, however, the severity of the incestuous abuse did not appear to be discriminative. This could be explained by the fact that the group of women who were interviewed in this study had in the majority of cases suffered from the severest kinds of incest, so there was not as much variation in this group as in other studies about incest, as in the study of Drayer [16].

The subjective reaction to the event (consisting of extreme anxiety combined with defense mechanisms of freezing and dissociation) appeared to be of major significance. This means that these events are so traumatic that the majority of women end up reacting in very similar ways. This could be explained by the theory of Janet [25]. He argued that the strong emotions aroused by traumatic events cause a disruption of the integrating faculties of the human mind, which lead to the development of symptoms later in life. ('L'émotion a une action dissolvante sur l'esprit, elle diminue la synthèse et le rend momentanément misérable' [26]). The events which cannot be integrated recur in nightmares and flashbacks. In the meantime the person has developed a coping style in which she reacts with numbness when confronted with stress. This could explain the emotional numbness and the amnesia which are parts of the avoidance symptoms of PTSD.

The last result of this study concerns the failure of diagnosing PTSD. It appeared that more than half (62%) of the women suffered from PTSD symptoms. This means that there is a great chance that an individual victim of incest will suffer from PTSD. This must be taken into account when dealing with the treatment of victims of incest. When treating these women, much can be learned from psychiatrists and physicians who have worked with victims of war [27].

Nevertheless, the odds are that this diagnosis will be missed, as a large range of other psychiatric symptoms may coincide. This could lead to the masking of their PTSD. These other symptoms are often of a very serious nature, such as self-destructive behavior, self-mutilation and suicidal tendencies. When confronted with these, psychiatrists may easily concentrate on the self-mutilation or suicide, as they will bring about acute crises and will require immediate intervention. Especially in institutional settings, the odds are that in those cases underlying PTSD symptoms will be overlooked.

This group of incest victims also displayed symptoms which were previously diagnosed as hysterical. These symptoms may lead to the failure in diagnosing PTSD for quite another reason: there is a tendency to regard hysterical women as unreliable [10]. Reports of former incest victims could therefore be easily dismissed as fantasies. In those cases, the diagnosis of PTSD will certainly be missed, as the first requirement for this diagnosis is the knowledge of the fact that the patient has experienced an identifiable traumatic event. If she is believed, however, her sexually provocative behavior (which 51 % of this group of incest victims displayed) may as yet lead to the misconception that she had provoked her own abuse. If this is the case, her posttraumatic symptoms, consisting of reexperiences, fear of men, avoidance of sexuality etc. will most certainly not be interpreted as a part of the posttraumatic Reexperiencing and Avoidance symptoms. From this study, it may be concluded that many victims of severe kinds of incest are suffering from PTSD. When dealing with an individual victim, therefore, it is important to think of PTSD as a diagnosis. Compared to other diagnoses, PTSD has the advantage of emphasizing not only mental, but also physical sequelae of traumatic events. Today women who claim that they have been victims of incest are generally believed. Despite this, the odds are that in some of these women the diagnosis of PTSD will be missed because they also display other psychiatric problems.

Acknowledgment

F.A. is a PhD student at the University of Amsterdam. W.E. is a PhD and Professor of Clinical Psychology at the University of Amsterdam. This study is based on a part of the research which is required for a doctoral dissertation about the psychiatric sequelae of sexual abuse of girls (incest). The research was done in the project 'Sexual child abuse and emotional phenomena' at the University of Amsterdam, in which B.J. Ensink took also part and which was supervised by W. Everaerd and N. Frijda.

References

1 Jacobson A, Richardson B: Assault experiences of 100 psychiatric inpatients: evidence of the need for routine inquiry. Am J Psychiatry 1987; 144:7:908–912.

2 Bagley C, Ramsay R: Sexual abuse in childhood: Psychososocial outcomes and implications for social work practice. Soc Work Pract Sex Prob 1985;4:33–47.

3 Carmen Hilberman E, Rieker Perri P, Mills T: Victims of violence and psychiatric illness. Am J Psychiatry 1984;141:3:378–383.

4 Brière J, Runz M: Post sexual abuse trauma; in Wyatt GE, Powell GJ (eds): Lasting Effects of Child Sexual Abuse. Beverley Hills, Sage, 1988, pp 85–99.

5 Walsh BW, Rosen PM: Self-Mutilation. Theory, Research and Treatment. New York, The Guilford Press, 1988.

6 Herman JL, Perry JC, van der Kolk B: Childhood trauma in borderline personality disorder. Am J Psychiatry 1989;146:4:490–495.

7 Morrison J: Childhood sexual histories of women with somatisation disorder. Am J Psychiatry 1989;146: 239–241.

8 Silbert MH, Pines AM: Sexual child abuse as an antecedent to prostitution. Int J Child Abuse Neglect 1981;5:400–411.

9 Terr LC: Childhood traumas: an outline and overview. Am J Psychiatry 1991;148:10–20.

10 Kraepelin E: Psychiatrie. Ein Lehrbuch für Studierende und Ärzte, vol 4, part III. Leipzig, Barth, 1915.

11 Van der Kolk B (ed): Psychological Trauma, Washington, American Psychiatric Press, 1987.

12 Lindberg FH, Distad LJ: 1985 Posttraumatic stress disorders in women who experienced childhood incest. Int J Child Abuse Neglect 1985;9: 329–334.

13 Donaldson M, Gardner R: Diagnosis and treatment of post traumatic stress among women after childhood incest; in Figley C (ed): Trauma and Its Wake. New York, Brunner/Mazel, 1985, vol 1, pp 356–377.

14 Lacoursière RB, Godfrey KE, Ruby LM: Traumatic neurosis in the etiology of alcoholism: Vietnam combat and other trauma. Am J Psychiatry 1980;137:966–968.

15 Russell DEH: The Secret Trauma. Incest in the Lives of Girls and Women. New York, Basic Books, 1986.

16 Drayer N: Seksuele traumatisering in de jeugd. Gevolgen op lange termijn van seksueel misbruik van meisjes door verwanten; thesis Amsterdam, 1990.
17 Browning D, Boatman B: Children at risk. Am J Psychiatry 1977;134: 69–72.
18 Horowitz MJ: Stress Response Syndromes. New York, Jason Aronson, 1976.
19 Kretschmer E: Hysteria, Reflex and Instinct. London, Owen, 1961.
20 Spiegel D: Dissociating damage. Am J Clin Hypnosis 1986;29:123–131.
21 Finkelhor D: Child Sexual Abuse. Theory and Research. New York, The Free Press, 1984.
22 American Psychiatric Association: Diagnostic and Statistical Manual of Mental Disorders, ed 3, revised. Washington, APA, 1987.
23 Keane TM, Caddel JM, Taylor KL: Mississippi scale for combat-related post-traumatic stress disorder: three studies in reliability and validity. J Consult Clin Psychol 1988;56:85–90.
24 Frenken J, van der Stolk B: Therapeuten en slachtoffers van incest. Deventer, van Loghum Slaterus, 1987.
25 Janet P: De l'angoisse à l'extase. Paris, Alcan, 1928.
26 Janet P: L'état mental des hystériques. Paris, Alcan, 1911, p 532.
27 Krystal H: Integration and Self-Healing: Affect, Trauma and Alexythymia. Hillsdale/New York, Analytic Press, 1988.

2nd Europ Conf on Traumatic Stress
Psychother Psychosom 1992;57:152–157

Dora Black[a]
Jean Harris-Hendriks[b]
Tony Kaplan[c]

[a] Royal Free Hospital School of Medicine, and
[b] Royal Free Hospital, London;
[c] Chase Farm Hospital, Enfield, and RFHSM, London, UK

Father Kills Mother: Post-Traumatic Stress Disorder in the Children

Key Words
Post-Traumatic Stress Disorders (PTSD)
Parental killing
Bereavement
Children
Murder
Grief
Adolescents
Treatment
Research

Abstract
Results of a study of over 100 children whose father killed their mother have been summarized and principles for practice have been formulated. All children orphaned by the death of one parent at the other's hands should be seen as soon as possible in a child psychiatry department and assessed. An immediate crisis intervention will probably be needed if they witnessed the killing to prevent PTSD. Bereavement counselling will be helpful in most cases. The caretakers will need support and help with their own mourning. Placement, access and custody, compensation, seeing the body, attending the funeral and dealing with family conflict will all need consideration. Long-term follow-up and further research are recommended.

Introduction

Children whose father kills their mother are orphaned by this act. Not only are they deprived of their mother by the catastrophe of her death, but also their father is suddenly absent, taken away to jail, or in a mental hospital, on the run or dead by his own hand. These are the children of a woman who dies a violent death and the children of the killer.

For child psychiatry teams these are difficult cases, and few individuals will have experience of working with more than one or two such families in a professional lifetime. As a result of the senior author's interest in bereaved children, many were referred in the first place for help with bereavement issues and we found ourselves with a uniquely large series of cases. We published our first paper in 1988 [1] and consequently were referred

Dr. Dora Black
Consultant Child Psychiatrist
Royal Free Hospital
London, NW3 2QG (UK)

0033–3190/92/
0574–0152$2.75/0

many more. To date we have seen personally 76 children and their caretakers, occasionally their jailed fathers, plus social workers, probation officers, grandparents etc. We have also seen 4 children whose mothers killed their fathers. We have information on 41 more cases whom we have not seen.

We estimate that in England and Wales, there are likely to be about 50 families a year, involving between 100 and 150 children who are affected. The plight of these children cannot be exaggerated. They are often witness to the killing, may be left alone with the dead body of their mother, may have to summon help or attempt to defend her. They may witness their father's subsequent suicide or defection, may be the only source of information for the police and social services who have to find relatives to care for them. They may have to give statements to the policc about what happened and later act as witnesses in court. They often lose, at one blow, their parents, their home, their toys, clothes and possessions, their friends, their school, their neighbours and even their siblings if, as is often the case with large families, different relatives each take one or two of the children.

What is even more important is that they lose their self-esteem. To be the child of a killer is not an enviable role. It cannot long be hidden, although the children we have seen, if they were not present at the killing (and sometimes even if they were), are the last to be told what happened to their parents. They and their carers may need professional advice and help with mourning and with the psychiatric sequelae that commonly develop. Where children should live and with whom, whether they should attend the funeral, see their father in prison, see the dead body of their mother are questions which require consideration and discussion. Some case examples may help to illustrate these points.

Case 1. Diana, aged 6 was the only child of separated, middle-class parents. After an access visit, father shot mother at point blank range and then rushed out of the house and committed suicide by crashing his car. Diana was left alone with the dead body of her mother. She tried to telephone the police, using the emergency number she had learned. Unfortunately she could not get through. At some time she must have fallen asleep and in the morning she tried again with success. The police came and were able to find a neighbour to look after her. No one in the neighbourhood knew where relatives lived but after a few days they were located in a city two hundred miles away. The elderly paternal grandparents took Diana to their home but found her too much of a handful. Mother's parents were also elderly and could not have her. D.B. was consulted by the grandparents 1 week after the death. Diana was seemingly unconcerned about recent events until invited to draw a picture.

She drew a man holding a gun, larger than the father himself, and the dead mother. Diana said when drawing her 'I can only draw a sad face, I can't draw a happy one'. Then she depicted the car crash of father. She said she had poured lemonade on mother to revive her and at this point began to sob uncontrollably, the first tears that her grandparents had seen since the death. They had, like most caretakers, avoided reminders of the parents and the tragedy and had given the child no opportunity to tell the story or to try to make sense of what had happened. This is a common finding.

Case 2. Maria was 4 when her father stabbed her mother who had announced her intention to leave him. Father then left the house and threw himself under a bus but survived, badly hurt. Maria was alone all night with the body. When seen by us a few days later she was living with mother's parents who found her difficult to manage and had not yet discussed the death with her. Maria could only talk about 'red water', presumably a reference to the blood she had seen. The grandparents and social worker asked us to help find out what Maria had experienced and to help explain what had happened. Using large dolls, we helped her aunt and grandparents tell her that her parents had had a big fight, and that daddy had hurt mummy with a knife. She had had to go to hospital but the doctors had not been able to make her better and she had died. We helped them to talk about what it meant for someone to die. That it was irreversible and that people looked different and could not talk or move, or eat any more. We arranged for her to see her dead mother with her aunt and our child psychiatric nurse, and to attend the funeral. We have seen her regularly since and have advised on placement. She has begun to talk about her knowledge of the knife hidden in the parents' room, her guilt at having told father about mother's lover and her desire for father to say he is sorry for what happened. She has visited her jailed father.

Case 3. Harry, aged 6, was referred with his 2 older sisters by social services for advice about access to father. Harry was invited to draw a picture. We were told by his uncle with whom he had lived since his mother was killed by his father that Harry did not know how mother died or where father was. Harry's picture indicates that he knew and may have witnessed the events as what he depicts was the truth. He shows the 3 children asleep in bed when his father hit his mother with an axe. Then his mother falls dead with blood around her shoulders. It also shows his reluctance to leave his own house for his uncle's (he has no legs and no face in the drawing) and it indicates that he has thought about visiting his father in jail.

There are many issues that arise in dealing with these cases of personal as opposed to mass disaster, some of which we have dealt with elsewhere [2]. In this paper we concentrate on two main issues, post-traumatic stress disorder (PTSD), and immediate management with consideration of preventive interventions.

Post-Traumatic Stress Disorder. There has been much controversy about this concept in adults and even more in children. Garmezey and Rutter [3], summarizing published studies on children and disaster concluded that in the majority of children exposed to severe stress, disturbances are short lived and a specific diagnostic category of PTSD is not needed for children. However, the literature surveyed did not include children experiencing a major disaster and Yule and Williams' [4] study of the child survivors of the ferry disaster in the English Channel led them to conclude that children do show intense and long-lasting behavioural disturbances in major disaster and that amnesia, intrusive thoughts and flashbacks can occur in quite young children. Terr [5], when she described her findings in the children kidnapped in the Chowchilla bus at a conference was ridiculed and denigrated. Benedek [6] describing this scene, concluded that 'the audience's response of disbelief, in the face of carefully collected documentation, might have been so intense because it was difficult for professionals to accept that traumatic events caused by fellow humans in the lives of children might colour and shape their lives for years to come'. Sugar [7] in his review concludes that most children have psychopathological reactions to disasters and these conclusions are echoed by Yule and by Parry-Jones [unpubl. data] in his study of the child survivors of Lockerbie. The change has come when the children themselves have been examined by child experts, rather than relying on adults', especially parents' reports. It is probable that the massive scale of the trauma and loss for the children overwhelms adults and makes them employ denial to protect the children and themselves. Terr [8] provides a comprehensive overview which indicates generally increased acceptance of this diagnostic concept.

We find that, in the cases we are describing, a mechanism of being appalled at the scale of the trauma to the children is active not only in the relatives but in the professionals who previously may not have come across such an event. An assessment of the presence and severity of PTSD needs to be made in every case, since, given the violence these children witness, it is likely that many will develop the syndrome. In our sample, nearly half the children had been present at the killing. Most of those present had symptoms of PTSD, whereas it was not found in those who were absent from home at the time of the killing. PTSD in children is discussed by Pynoos et al. [9]. They define PTSD in children following DSM III [10], as follows: (1) occurrence of a distressing, traumatic event; (2) repetitive re-experiencing of the event in play, dreams, intrusive images and sounds; (3) psychic numbing or affective constriction; (4) incident-specific phenomena that were previously not present (startle reactions, avoidant behaviour, sleep disturbances, etc.). DSM III R [11] substantially is similar but allows formal diagnosis of PTSD only after 1 month subsequent to the traumatic event.

In those children who are traumatized by witnessing the killing, normal grieving may be inhibited [12] and other factors may also inhibit this process. The child may feel compelled to remain silent because of shame or because he may wish to protect others from the intense feelings of horror, rage, sadness and powerlessness which his story may provoke. This suppression is particularly likely if his carers are kin, since they will be more emotionally affected by the child's account. The child may learn from the carers that it is wrong to talk about what he knows or that it is in some way dangerous. We know that mourning cannot begin until death is made real. Part of the assessment must be to ascertain what the child has been told, and what he knows (which may be quite different), and at what stage of understanding about the permanence of death he has reached. We know from the work of Lansdown and Benjamin [13], amongst others, that even young children can have a good understanding of the main components of the concept of death.

Relatives are more likely than unrelated carers to decide not to tell the children the true nature of their mother's death. Of the children who were not told, 70% were living with kin. Without this knowledge the children will have difficulty in understanding their changed circumstances and the reactions of those around them and may not be able to effectively mourn their losses.

Identifying Psychiatric Disorder. Other disorders are common. Excluding PTSD, we found over half the children had one or more other psychiatric problems, and only 10% had no problems at all.

Placement, Custody and Access. Placement after the death is very problematic. Half the children went to kin but many of these placements broke down, because of the grief of the relatives, or because of the pressures heaped upon the children by the relatives' antagonism for the other side. If the children go to maternal relatives they rarely see their father and their fantasies about his power and capacity for evil may become very frightening. If they go to father's relatives, the relatives see it as their duty to justify father's actions. The mother is often reviled and denigrated. The implication often is that she brought her killing on herself. Paternal relatives may also keep the child *for* father on his release, consequently making it difficult for him or her to form a permanent attachment. Brinich [14] has suggested that when relatives become parents by default the dynamics of the relationship often are different from voluntary assumption of parenthood. Involuntary parents both over-protect and subtly reject their foster-child.

Management and Treatment

Clinical experience has shown that crisis intervention limits the severity of post-traumatic stress symptoms [1, 8, 15–17] although this needs confirmation by controlled trials. This approach depends on helping the child to recount the traumatic events and his feelings and integrate them in as comprehensive a way as possible. When we see the children soon after the killing, in addition to individual assessment, we involve the child or children in sibling/group therapy. This is a modified form of family therapy, in which the caretaker may be included or may have separate counselling depending on the relationship and the issues identified at assessment. Unrelated foster-parents appreciate help with management. Maternal relatives may need, in addition, help with their own mourning, and work on their anger and resentment. Their own children may have to make many adaptations to accommodate the needy bereaved children and some family therapy is useful. Much of our therapeutic work is at a cognitive level, helping the child to understand what has been experienced.

This work is very difficult and can be exhausting. In our experience, prevention or amelioration of post-traumatic stress symptoms is possible if the children are seen early. We have found that children are very willing to tell us what happened and indeed are relieved that someone wishes to know. Often this leads to a compulsive repetition of the events which caretakers find embarrassing. It may be necessary to repeat this work over time, according to each child's age and understanding, an additional burden for adult carers who must work through their own grief.

Case 5. Two girls aged 3 and 5 were present at their mother's killing. The older one developed asthma subsequently, which dramatically came on when painting a picture of a rainbow at the seventh therapeutic session. The therapist recognized that the asthma which accompanied her attempts was the sound the girl had heard as her mother attempted to take in air with a cut throat. The child's symptoms were relieved by interpretation.

Case 6. Larry, aged 5 had night terrors every night following the death of his father at his mother's hands when both were drunk. He had witnessed the killing and had stayed all night with mother and the body of his father until mother, sober the next morning gave herself up to the police after taking Larry to her sister's. Using the technique described by Lask [18] of waking the child just before the night terror usually began, he was cured within a few days. He is having psychotherapy to help him with his grief and other symptoms, and the maternal aunt values the help given. Thus, timely interpretation and relevant behavioural techniques can relieve symptoms and facilitate longer term interventions. Early intervention is economic and effective.

Principles for Practice

As a result of our experience with these troubled children we have formulated the following recommendations.

Immediately after the Killing. (1) Placement should be with familiar people, who will need immediate advice and support. (2) Custody decisions are required at once. Preferably the State should act as parent while plans are formulated. The children may require independent legal representation and advocacy. (3) Primary health care services should be alerted about the children and early consultations sought from child mental health services with particular reference to assessment of PTSD and the need for crisis intervention or other treatment. Expert advice should be sought regarding the planning of access to father and key relatives, the desirability of seeing the body and of attending the funeral.

In the Longer Term. (1) Permanent placement planning should begin as soon as possible and should certainly not be delayed pending the outcome of father's trial. The emergency placement should not become permanent by default. (2) The decisions about access and custody must be guided by the principle of the child's best interests. In particular the right of the child to have contact with father must be borne in mind. We recommend that the child should see the father at least once in prison to reduce the likelihood of frightening fantasies about his power. (3) Therapeutic help should be available as needed. Crisis intervention and bereavement counselling are likely to be needed by all children who witnessed the killing. (4) Decisions about whether the children are fit to give witness in court at their father's trial must be made by experts. If it is essential that the child does so, he must be supported by someone experienced in anticipating what problems may arise and preparing the child for the experience. The child will probably need post-trial counselling. (5) Consideration must be given to obtaining compensation for the children where appropriate, safeguarding their inheritance, obtaining maintenance from their father, or the State, and to protecting them from family conflict and pressures to side with maternal or paternal relatives. This may mean removing them from a placement with kin if antagonism is harming them. (6) Long-term studies are needed to ascertain what happens to these children, especially when they are returned to their father, and when they grow up. Comparative studies of different treatments are needed.

References

1 Black D, Kaplan T: Father kills mother. Issues and problems encountered by a child psychiatric team. Br J Psychiatry 1988;153: 624–630.
2 Black D, Kaplan T, Harris Hendriks J: Father kills mother: Effects on the children; in Wilson J, Raphael B (eds): International Handbook of Traumatic Stress Syndromes. New York, Plenum Press, 1992.
3 Garmezey N, Rutter M: Acute reactions to stress, in Rutter M, Hersov L (eds): Child and Adolescent Psychiatry: Modern Approaches. Oxford, Blackwell, 1985.
4 Yule W, Williams R: Post-traumatic stress reactions in children. J Trauma Stress 1990;3:279–295.
5 Terr LC: Children Traumatized in Small Groups; in Eth S, Pynoos RS (eds): Post-Traumatic Stress Disorder in Children. Washington, APA, 1985, pp 45–70.
6 Benedek EP: Children and psychic trauma: A brief review of contemporary thinking; in Eth S, Pynoos RS (eds): Post-Traumatic Stress Disorder in Children. Washington, APA, 1985, pp 1–17.
7 Sugar M: Children in a disaster: an overview. Child Psychiatry Hum Dev 1989;19:163–179.
8 Terr LC: Childhood traumas – an outline and overview. Am J Psychiatry 1991;148:10–20.
9 Pynoos RS, Frederick C, Nader K, Arroyo W, et al: Life threat and posttraumatic stress in school-age children. Annual Meeting of the American Psychiatric Association (1985, Dallas, Texas). Arch Gen Psychiatry 1987;44:1057–1063.
10 American Psychiatric Association: Diagnostic and Statistical Manual of Mental Disorders. Washington, APA, 1980.
11 American Psychiatric Association: Diagnostic and Statistical Manual of Mental Disorders. Washington, APA, 1987.
12 Eth, S, Pynoos RS: Interaction of trauma and grief in childhood; in Eth S, Pynoos RS (eds): Post-Traumatic Stress Disorder in Children. Washington, APA, 1985, pp 169–186.
13 Lansdown R, Benjamin G: The development of the concept of death in children aged 5–9 years. Child Care Health Dev 1985;11:13–20.
14 Brinich PM: Love and anger in relatives who 'adopt' orphaned children: Parents by default. Bereavement Care 1989;8:14–16.
15 Pynoos RS, Eth S: Witness to violence: The child interview. J Am Acad Child Psychiatry 1986;25: 306–319.
16 Ayalon O: Coping with terrorism; in Herchenbaum D, Jememki ME (eds): Stress Reduction and Prevention. New York, Plenum Press, 1983.
17 Yule W: The effects of disasters on children. Assoc Child Psychol Psychiatry 1989;11:6:3–6.
18 Lask B: Novel and non-toxic treatment for night terrors. Br Med J 1988;297:592.

2nd Europ Conf on Traumatic Stress
Psychother Psychosom 1992;57:158–163

Marc De Boer [a]
Wybrand Op den Velde [a]
Paul J.R. Falger [b]
Johannes E. Hovens [c]
Johannes H.M. De Groen [d]
Hans Van Duijn [b]

[a] Department of Psychiatry, St. Lucas Hospital, Amsterdam;
[b] Department of Medical Psychology, University of Limburg School of Medicine, Maastricht;
[c] Centrum 45, National Center for the treatment of World War II victims, Oegstgeest;
[d] Department of Clinical Neurophysiology, University of Limburg School of Medicine, Maastricht;
[e] Department of Clinical Neurophysiology, St. Lucas Hospital, Amsterdam, The Netherlands

Fluvoxamine Treatment for Chronic PTSD: A Pilot Study

Key Words
Posttraumatic stress disorder, chronic
Pharmacotherapy
Fluvoxamine

Abstract

A group of 24 Dutch World War II Resistance veterans with a documented traumatic war history and a (partially) positive diagnosis of current posttraumatic stress disorder (PTSD) was studied. This special group of war victims is characterised by chronicity, suffering from intractable posttraumatic complaints for decades. They were treated with fluvoxamine (Fevarin), a selective serotonin reuptake inhibitor with antidepressive and anxiolytic properties. The study was designed as an open-ended, outpatient pilot study, with a treatment period of 12 weeks. Results of clinical examination, and questionnaires investigating PTSD, depression, sleeping problems, anxiety, and vital exhaustion indicate that a significant number of the subjects improved with respect to their PTSD symptomatology, and their symptoms of anxiety and vital exhaustion. However, at the end of the study, quantitative improvement was modest. The results indicate that treatment with fluvoxamine may offer alleviation of chronic PTSD symptoms, in particular insomnia, nightmares, anxiety, intrusive recollections, guilt feelings and tiredness.

Introduction

Relatively few studies have been published on the pharmacological treatment of posttraumatic stress disorder (PTSD) [1–4]. With respect to antidepressants, some promising results have been reported on MAO inhibitors [5–9], and tricyclic antidepressants [9–15]. Preliminary reports concerning treatment of PTSD with fluoxetine show favorable results [16, 17]. The selective serotonin (5-hydroxytryptamine; 5-HT) reuptake inhibitor fluvoxamine (Fevarin) has been shown to be an effective antidepressant [18–20]. In addition, in several studies anxiolytic activity of fluvoxamine has been reported in the treatment of the anxiety disorders, obsessive compulsive disorder (OCD) [21–23], and panic disorder

M. De Boer, MD
Department of Psychiatry
St. Lucas Hospital
Amsterdam (The Netherlands)

0033–3190/92/
0574–0158$2.75/0

(PD) [24]. Though a useful concept, PTSD contains a broad variety of symptoms overlapping with major depressive disorders (MDD) and anxiety disorders. As a consequence of this overlapping symptomatology, it is of interest to explore the effects of fluvoxamine in PTSD. Fluvoxamine is a specific and potent 5-HT uptake inhibitor, structurally different from the tricyclic antidepressants, with virtually no effect on noradrenergic, dopaminergic, histaminergic or muscarine receptors [25]. In this open-ended, nonclinical pilot study, we studied the clinical efficacy of fluvoxamine in a group of elderly patients suffering from chronic PTSD.

Methods

Subjects. Forty subjects, invited by letter, participated in this study. All subjects were former members of the Dutch Resistance during World War II, and had an impartially documented history of excessive war stress. Most of them participated in an earlier study on war stress [26, 27]. In several respects these war victims constitute an extraordinary group.

The majority had been suffering from posttraumatic complaints for several decades and has learned 'to live with their problems'. Most of them received a special War Veterans Pension because of their mental problems. In the long course of their illness, many of them had consulted a number of professionals and had gradually lost any hope to find a cure. Others had a long history of psychoactive drugs use, in particular benzodiazepines, without satisfactory outcome. Their motivation to participate in the present treatment study was, generally speaking, poor. Most of them did not expect a positive outcome for their own personal well-being, but were nevertheless willing to participate for the benefit of the scientific results for other war victims.

Procedure. After obtaining informed consent, a psychiatric examination was carried out to establish current PTSD, according to the DSM-III-R criteria. This was performed by means of the Dutch translation [Koster van Groos, 1986, unpubl. manuscript] of the SCID-R PTSD module [28]. In case a subject did not meet all criteria for PTSD, she or he was included if a sufficient number of complaints of either the intrusive or avoidance symptom clusters was present (partial PTSD). Subjects with mental retardation, severe alcohol abuse, psychotic features, and obvious signs of organic brain disorder were excluded. A general physical examination was performed, followed by ECG and laboratory investigations. In order to avoid possible complications, subjects with risk factors, such as relevant cardiovascular disease, and endocrine disturbances were also excluded.

Of the 40 subjects willing to participate, 29 (73%) had a positive or partial positive diagnosis of PTSD. After the initial interview, 4 of the latter refrained from participation. One subject was excluded because of severe cardiac disease. Thus, 24 subjects entered the study.

All psychotropics, except for benzodiazepines, were terminated at least two weeks prior to the start of the 12-week study period. Fluvoxamine was administered in weekly rising doses, up to 300 mg daily. The current dosis was adjusted on observed effects and side effects in weekly telephone consultations during the first 4 weeks of the study.

Instruments. Severity of psychiatric symptoms was assessed by means of: (1) the Global Clinical Impression Scale (GCI); (2) the Zung Depression Scale (Zung) [29]; (3) the Dutch adaptation of the Spielberger State/Trait Anxiety Inventory [30]; (4) a subscale of the Dutch Subjective Sleep Grading Scale, assessing sleep quality of the last night [31]; (5) a Dutch PTSD self-rating scale, measuring severity of PTSD symptoms [Hovens, unpubl. data]; (6) the Maastricht Questionnaire on vital exhaustion (MQ). This Dutch questionnaire purports to measure manifestations of vital exhaustion, a state characterized by feelings of unusual tiredness and general malaise [32, 33]. These rating scales were chosen because of their proven correlation with severity of symptoms of PTSD in earlier studies [34]. For all subjects who participated in the study, Spearman correlation coefficients were calculated for all questionnaire scores. These correlations were highly significant ($p < 0.005$), which indicates that the questionnaires are not independent in assessing symptomatology. These self-report rating scales, together with the GCI scale were taken at the beginning of the study, at 4 weeks, and at the end of the study period (in principle) at 12 weeks. Questionnaire results were analysed after a minimal participation of 4 weeks. In case subjects dropped out prematurely, the last observations were taken as end-study measurements (last observation carried forward method).

Statistical analysis was performed with the Wilcoxon matched-pairs signed-rank test.

Table 1. Rating scale results at week 4 and weeks 4–12, compared with baseline

	Week	Improved	Unchanged	Worse	p
GCI	4	9	6	0	0.008
	7–12	8	7	2	0.28
MQ	4	11	2	3	0.04
	7–12	11	3	3	0.04
PTSD self-rating	4	12	0	4	0.03
	7–12	12	1	4	0.05
State anxiety	4	11	2	3	0.09
	7–12	10	1	6	0.08
Trait anxiety	4	9	2	5	0.36
	7–12	13	1	3	0.008
Sleep last night	4	11	0	5	0.11
	7–12	11	0	6	0.20
Zung depression	4	8	3	5	0.30
	7–12	10	2	5	0.50

Results

Nine subjects terminated the study prematurely because of gastrointestinal complaints. One subject's sleep deteriorated and another 3 subjects discontinued the study because of physical complaints, which apparently were not related to fluvoxamine. A total of 11 subjects (46%) completed the full study, and 6 subjects terminated the study at 4–9 weeks. Thus, 17 subjects completed a treatment period of at least 4 weeks. Significant differences on the rating scales between the subjects who actually finished (n = 11) the study, and those who did not (n = 13) could not be demonstrated (Mann-Whitney U-Wilcoxon rank sum W test, p values 0.19–0.84).

Table 1 reports the results on the various rating scales in terms of experienced change. As can be seen, the majority of the subjects improved on the self-rating lists. At 4 weeks, the reported change towards improvement attains significance on vital exhaustion (the MQ) and the PTSD self-rating scale (p = 0.04 and 0.03, respectively). At 12 weeks, these changes attain significance on the MQ, the PTSD self-rating scale and the Trait anxiety scale (p = 0.04, 0.05 and 0.008 respectively). Trends towards improvement are shown with respect to State anxiety at week 4 and week 12 (p = 0.09 and 0.08, respectively). The interviewer-rated GCI shows significant improvement at 4 weeks (p = 0.008). At the end of the study, however, the number of subjects that did not change or worsened on the GCI exceeds the number of subjects that improved on this scale. The scores of the 3 questionnaires that show significant improvement at 12 weeks on the Wilcoxon matched-pairs signed-rank test are presented in figure 1.

As can been seen in the scores on trait anxiety, vital exhaustion, and PTSD the clinical efficacy of fluvoxamine is modest. A further analysis of the PTSD symptom profiles on the PTSD self-rating scale shows that those subjects with an improved PTSD rating (n = 12) reported a decrease of their feelings of survival guilt, insomnia, nightmares, intrusive recollections, explosiveness and fear. The other items showed less marked changes. Finally, after completion of the study period, 5 subjects insisted on continuation of the use of fluvoxamine.

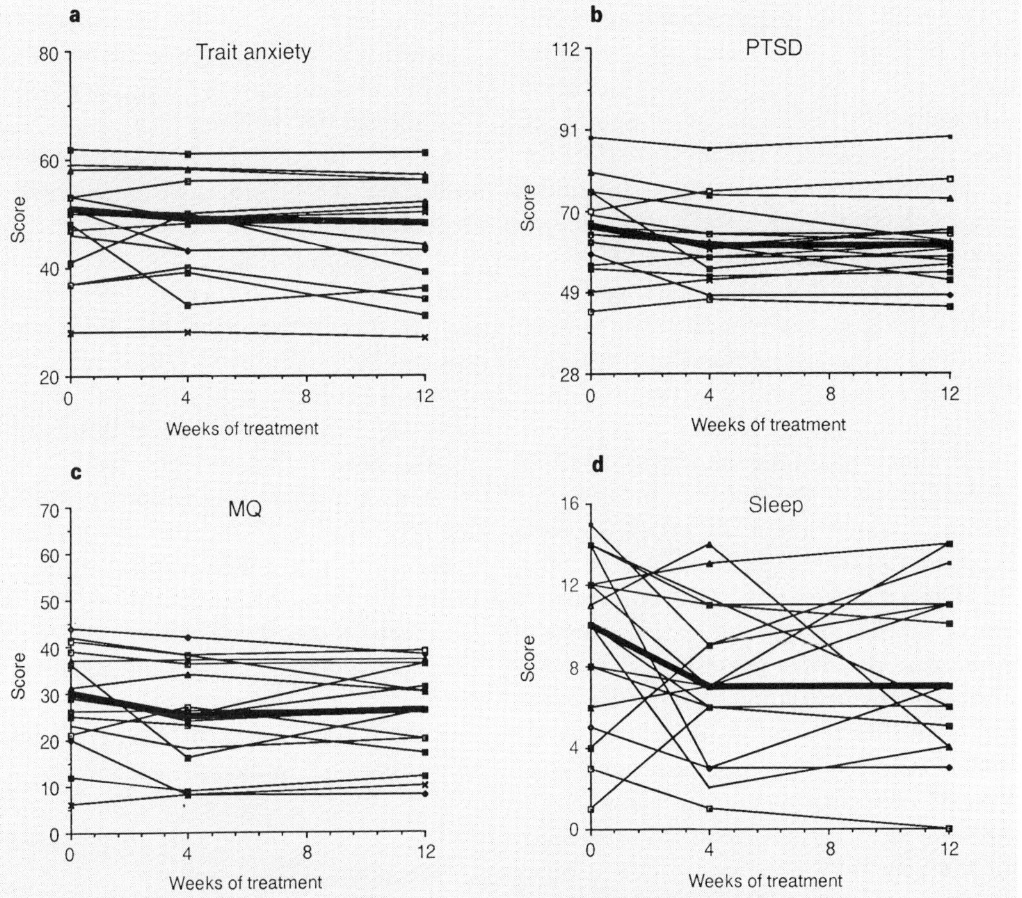

Fig. 1. Scores on the Trait anxiety (**a**), PTSD (**b**), MQ (**c**) self-rating, and sleep (**d**) scales plotted against study duration. The heavy line reflects the median.

Discussion

A significant number of the subjects improved with respect to their PTSD symptomatology, and the scores on anxiety, and vital exhaustion. However, quantitative improvement at the end of the study was slight. None of the subjects became free of PTSD symptoms. Although fluvoxamine is an antidepressant, and many subjects were depressed, the scores on the Zung depression scale did not show a significant improvement. A number of factors may account for the apparently modest efficacy of fluvoxamine in this group of PTSD sufferers. PTSD as a syndrome contains a broad variety of target symptoms for pharmacotherapy. Depressed Vietnam War combat veterans with frequent, explosive outbursts of rage, showed considerable improvement when treated with the 5-HT uptake inhibitor fluoxetine (Prozac) [16]. Yet, they differ greatly from the present, much older group, in which explosiveness is not predominant.

In contrast to most studies of antidepressants and anxiolytics, the present study was not applied to subjects seeking treatment. Most of them were in a stationary phase of their chronic World War II related PTSD. In several instances they only participated just for the expected benefit for other war victims. According to clinical impression as well as to the scores on the self-rating lists many of them were only moderately ill.

More than half of the subjects dropped out before the end of the study. Compared with studies on fluvoxamine in MDD, PD and OCD [18–24] these figures are high. A possible explanation for this could be a relative lack of motivation to sustain side effects of the medication in this moderately ill group.

An interesting finding with respect to the various PTSD self-rating scale items is the marked decrease in feelings of survival guilt. A possible explanation for this change may be the mere effect of participating in this study for the benefit of other war victims, which may have served as a counterbalance for their guilt feelings. The marked positive effect in the PTSD self-rating scale on DSM-III-R cluster B and D symptoms (intrusiveness and hyperarousal) and the scanty effect on avoidance symptoms (cluster C) is congruent with earlier findings [5, 6, 9, 12, 13]. In a recent study, though, amitryptiline appeared better than placebo with respect to the avoidance subscale of the Impact of Event Scale [15].

Although the statistical analysis of the entire group revealed only modest improvement, 5 of the 11 subjects who completed a treatment period of 12 weeks reported a substantial improvement of their overall condition. A further scrutiny of this subgroup showed that in particular their sleep quality was markedly improved. These subjects insisted on a continued use of fluvoxamine.

It may be concluded that in this group of elderly, chronic patients not seeking treatment, several distressing symptoms of PTSD could be alleviated by treatment with fluvoxamine. Although a great variety in the individual reactions was observed, several subjects reported a decrease of insomnia, anxiety, tiredness, nightmares, and guilt feelings. Five subjects in this study showed a marked improvement, which was of substantial subjective importance to them.

Acknowledgements

This study was supported by grants awarded from the Stichting 1940–1945, Amsterdam; Stichting Dienstverlening Verzetsdeelnemers, Dirkshorn; and Duphar Nederland BV, Amsterdam, the Netherlands. We are grateful to W.S. de Loos, MD, PhD for the referral of patients.

References

1 Van der Kolk BA: The drug treatment of post-traumatic stress disorder. J Affective Disord 1987;13:203–213.
2 Friedman MJ: Towards a rational pharmacotherapy for posttraumatic stress disorder: an interim report. Am J Psychiatry 1988;145:281–285.
3 Davidson JR, Nemeroff CB: Pharmacotherapy in posttraumatic stress disorder: Historical and clinical considerations and future directions. Psychopharmacol Bull 1989;25:422–425.
4 Schwartz L: A biopsychosocial treatment approach to posttraumatic stress disorder. J Trauma Stress 1990;3:221–238.
5 Hogben GL, Cornfield RB: Treatment of traumatic war neuroses with phenelzine. Arch Gen Psychiatry 1981;38:440–445.

6 Walker JI: Chemotherapy of traumatic war stress. Milit Med 1982; 147:1029–1033.
7 Cornfield R: Traumatic war neuroses: Some pharmacologic and psychophysiologic observations; in Schwartz H (ed): Psychotherapy of the Combat Veteran. Lancaster, MTP Press, 1984, pp 221–251.
8 Davidson J, Walker JI, Kilts C: A pilot study of phenelzine in the treatment of post-traumatic stress disorder. Br J Psychiatry 1987;150: 252–255.
9 Frank JB, Kosten TR, Giller EL, Dan E: A randomized clinical trial of phenelzine and imipramine for posttraumatic stress disorder. Am J Psychiatry 1988;145:1289–1291.
10 Burstein A: Treatment of post traumatic stress disorder with imipramine. Psychosomatics 1984;25: 681–686.
11 Falcon S, Ryan C, Chamberlain K, Curtis G: Tricyclics: Possible treatment for posttraumatic stress disorder. J Clin Psychiatry 1985;46:385–389.
12 Boehnlein JK, Kinzie JD, Ben R, Fleck J: One-year follow-up study of posttraumatic stress disorder among survivors of Cambodian Concentration camps. Am J Psychiatry 1985; 142:956–959.
13 Blake DJ: Treatment of acute posttraumatic stress disorder with tricyclic antidepressants. South Med J 1986;79:201–204.
14 Reist C, Kauffmann CD, Haier RJ, Sangdahl C, DeMet EM, Chicz-DeMet A, Nelson JN: A controlled trial of desipramine in 18 men with posttraumatic stress disorder. Am J Psychiatry 1989;146:513–516.
15 Davidson J, Kudler H, Smith R, Mahorney SL, Lipper S, Hammett E, Saunders WB, Cavenar JO: Treatment of posttraumatic stress disorder with Amitriptyline and placebo. Arch Gen Psychiatry 1990;47: 259–266.
16 Shay J: Fluoxetine reduces explosiveness and elevates mood of Vietnam combats vets with PTSD. J Trauma Stress, 1992;5:97–100.
17 Davidson J, Roth S, Newman E: Fluoxetine in posttraumatic stress disorder. J Trauma Stress 1991;4: 419–423.
18 Feighner JP, Boyer WF, Meredith CH, Hendrickson GG: A placebo-controlled inpatient comparison of fluvoxamine maleate and imipramine in major depression. Int Clin Psychopharmacol 1989;4:239–244.
19 De Jonghe F, Swinkels J, Tuynman-Qua H: Randomized double-blind study of fluvoxamine and maprotiline in treatment of depression. Pharmacopsychiatry 1991;24:21–27.
20 Martin AJ, Tebbs VM, Ashford JJ: Affective disorders in general practice. Treatment of 6000 patients with fluvoxamine. Pharmacotherapeutica 1987;5:40–49.
21 Goodman WK, Lawrence HP, Rasmussen SA, Delgado PL, Heninger GR, Charney DS: Efficacy of Fluvoxamine in obsessive-compulsive disorder. Arch Gen Psychiatry 1989;46:36–44.
22 Price HP, Goodman WK, Charney DS, Rasmussen SA, Heninger GR: Treatment of severe obsessive-compulsive disorder with fluvoxamine. Am J Psychiatry 1987;44:1059–1061.
23 Perse TL, Greist JH, Jefferson JW, Rosenfeld R, Dar R: Fluvoxamine treatment of obsessive-compulsive disorder. Am J Psychiatry 1987;144: 1543–1548.
24 Den Boer JA, Westenberg HG: Effect of a serotonin and noradrenaline uptake inhibitor in panic disorder; a double-blind comparative study with fluvoxamine and maprotiline. Int Clin Psychopharmacol 1988;3:59–74.
25 Claassen V: Review of the animal pharmacology and pharmacokinetics of fluvoxamine. Br J Clin Pharmacol 1983;15:349–355.
26 Op den Velde W, Falger PR, De Groen JHM, Van Duijn H, Hovens JE, Meijer P, Soons M, Schouten EG: Current psychiatric complaints of Dutch Resistance veterans from World War II. J Trauma Stress 1990;3:351–358.
27 Op den Velde W, Falger PR, Hovens JE, De Groen JHM, Lasschuit LJ, Van Duijn H, Schouten EG: PTSD in Dutch Resistance veterans from World War II; in Wilson JP, Rafael B (eds): The International Handbook of Traumatic Stress Syndromes. New York, Plenum Press, in press.
28 Spitzer R, Williams J, Gibbon M: Instruction Manual for the Structured Clinical Interview for DSM-III-R. 1985, Nonpatient Version (SCID-NP-V). New York, Biometrics Research Department.
29 Dijkstra P: De zelfbeoordelingsschaal van depressie van Zung (The Zung depression self assessment scale); in Van Praag HM, Rooymans HG (eds): Stemming en ontstemming. Amsterdam, Bohn, 1974.
30 Van der Ploeg HM: Handleiding bij de zelfbeoordelings vragenlijst (Manual for the self-rating scale). Lisse, Zwets & Zeitlinger, 1979.
31 De Graaf W: Huisarts en slaapgedrag. Waarnemingen omtrent slaapgedrag van patienten in een huisartsenpraktijk; PhD thesis, University of Amsterdam, 1984.
32 Appels A, Höppener P, Mulder P: A questionnaire to assess premonitory symptoms of myocardial infarction. Int J Cardiol 1987;17:15–24.
33 Falger PJ, Op den Velde W, Hovens JE, Schouten EG, De Groen JHM, Van Duyn H: Current post traumatic stress disorder and cardiovascular disease: Indicators in Dutch resistance veterans from World War II. Psychother Psychosom 1992;57:164–171.
34 Kauffman CD, Reist C, Djenderedjian A, Nelson JN, Haier RJ: Biological markers of affective disorders and posttraumatic stress disorder: A pilot study with desipramine. J Clin Psychiatry 1987;48:366–367.

2nd Europ Conf on Traumatic Stress
Psychother Psychosom 1992;57:164–171

Paul R.J. Falger[a]
Wybrand Op den Velde[b]
Johannes E. Hovens[b]
Erik G.W. Schouten[a]
Johannes H.M. De Groen[c]
Hans Van Duijn[d]

Departments of
[a] Medical Psychology and
[c] Clinical Neurophysiology,
University of Limburg School of Medicine, Maastricht, and
Departments of
[b] Psychiatry and
[d] Clinical Neurophysiology,
St. Lucas Hospital, Amsterdam,
The Netherlands

Current Posttraumatic Stress Disorder and Cardiovascular Disease Risk Factors in Dutch Resistance Veterans from World War II

Key Words
Resistance veterans
Posttraumatic stress disorder
Type A behavior
Life stressors
Vital exhaustion
DSM-III
DSM-III-R
Structured clinical interview
Clinical rating interview

Abstract

The extraordinary trauma experienced by Resistance veterans from World War II (WW II) and other veterans may be associated with an increased incidence of posttraumatic stress disorder (PTSD) and somatic morbidity, including cardiovascular disease (CVD). This study explored some relationships between current PTSD and CVD risk factors in 147 male Dutch WW II Resistance veterans. They were compared to 65 same-aged male patients with a recent myocardial infarction and 79 surgical patients. Of these subjects, WW II Resistance veterans scored highest on CVD risk factors (i.e., angina pectoris, type A behavior, life stressors, and vital exhaustion), except smoking. Fifty-six percent of these veterans were currently suffering from PTSD. They reported CVD risk factors, in particular type A behavior and vital exhaustion, more often than veterans without PTSD; they also reported more premorbid adverse living conditions. These data suggest that early sensitization to environmental stressors may be associated with a high prevalence of current PTSD and excess CVD risk factors in subjects exposed to extraordinary war-time trauma and that this may lead to vital exhaustion.

Introduction

The Nazi occupation of the Netherlands (1940–1945) met with little organized resistance. At most, some 5% of the adult population either supported or actually took part in the Dutch Resistance at any time during World War II (WW II) [1]. Resistance activities included aid to persons in hiding (mostly Jews and members of the Allied Air Forces

Paul R.J. Falger, PhD, Department of Medical Psychology
University of Limburg School of Medicine
Cardiovascular Research Institute Maastricht
PO Box 616, NL–6200 MD Maastricht (The Netherlands)

0033–3190/92/
0574–0164$2.75/0

who had crashed over occupied territory), the illegal dissemination of news about the Netherlands or occupied Europe as antidote to the Nazi propaganda, espionage, and acts of sabotage; armed resistance was carried out on a limited scale. When Resistance members got caught, which happened frequently, they were interrogated, imprisoned in labor or concentration camps where most of them succumbed, or executed. Therefore, the war experiences of surviving Resistance veterans are different from those of Korean, Vietnam, and Middle Eastern war veterans. Participation in the Resistance implied living under constant pressure and the perpetual fear of being betrayed, and its possible consequences of imprisonment or death.

In the postwar years, the regularly available medical attention for these veterans was directed at somatic health sequelae [2]. Behavioral and psychic reactions were seen as temporary and were expected to disappear spontaneously. As a result, these veterans did not always receive optimum medical or psychiatric care and, until recently, only a few studies were conducted on their medical condition to date. However, it has now become evident that the extraordinary trauma experienced by Resistance and other war veterans may be associated with an increased incidence of posttraumatic stress disorder (PTSD) [3, 4] and somatic morbidity [5, 6], including cardiovascular disease (CVD) [7, 8].

This long-term failure to recognize the origin of their health problems seems to have contributed to the chronic feelings of general mistrust characteristically found among aging Resistance veterans and may have impaired their ability to cope with their traumatic experiences during and since WW II. In fact, their complaints about chronic sleep disturbances and malaise was the reason we decided to conduct the present survey [9]. We had observed earlier that those symptoms were associated with signs of PTSD and with 'vital exhaustion', both physical and psychological. 'Vital exhaustion' has been described as a psychological state characterized by feelings of unusual tiredness, general malaise, and irritability [10]. Several studies have shown that exhaustion, or aspects of it, constitutes a strong risk for myocardial infarction (MI), independent of other risk factors [11–14]. This risk is of about the same magnitude as that associated with smoking, but larger than that conferred by psychosocial risk factors such as type A behavior [12, 13]. Therefore, we explored the relationships between current PTSD, 'vital exhaustion', and a number of CVD risk factors in Dutch Resistance veterans from WW II.

Subjects and Methods

As Dutch Resistance veterans of WW II never had been registered formally, all of the 813 male veterans between 60 and 65 years of age as of January 1, 1986, listed with the Dutch 'Stichting (foundation) 1940–1945', were invited to participate. These veterans were between 15 and 24 years old at any time during WW II. Because of their age, they were supposedly more vulnerable to extraordinary war trauma than older veterans [15]. From this population, a representative sample of 147 veterans was drawn [2]. Their objectively and impartially documented Resistance records indicate that 50% had been engaged in the Resistance for up to 2 years, 16% for 2–3 years, and 34% for more than 3 years. Subsequently, half of these veterans had been arrested and incarcerated in Nazi prisons and forced labor and death camps, mostly until the end of the war.

These 147 veterans were compared to 65 male patients with a recent MI and 79 male surgical patients of about the same age. Those patients had participated in a previous study on sleep complaints, behavioral characteristics, 'vital exhaustion', life stressors, and first MI [12, 13].

All 291 subjects completed a number of questionnaires, namely the Maastricht Questionnaire and the Rose Questionnaire, assessing current 'vital exhaus-

Table 1. Cardiovascular disease risk factors in WW II Resistance veterans, heart patients, and surgical patients

Variables	RV (n = 147)	HP (n = 65)	Sur (n = 79)	p
Mean age	64.1	61.3	61.0	
SD	1.5	4.3	4.1	
Angina pectoris, %	31	26	7	*
Smoking, %	55	82	60	*
Type A behavior, %	82	60	51	*
Mean 'vital exhaustion'[1]	23.6	17.9	12.9	*
SD	12.7	12.0	9.7	
Mean life stressors[2]	3.8	3.4	2.5	*
SD	1.9	2.5	1.5	

RV: Resistance veterans; HP: heart patients; SP: surgical patients.
* $p < 0.001$.
[1] MQ 21 items.
[2] 12 life stressors.

tion' and angina pectoris, respectively, and the Life Styles Questionnaire about current adverse health habits [12, 13]. Next, they were interviewed with the Structured Interview, assessing type A behavior [16], and with the Biographical Interview about life stressors over the life-span as employed in the previous study [13]. These stressors included stressful experiences from (a) childhood and adolescence, such as prolonged financial problems and familial conflicts at home; (b) work, for instance prolonged conflicts with supervisors and subordinates, or unemployment, and (c) family and social life, such as prolonged marital conflicts or educational problems with children. Stressors associated with WW II were, however, *not* included in the Biographical Interview, since the previous study focused on normative life stressors that were expected to have occurred in at least 10% of the participants [13]. In a pilot study, particular war-related stessors had been reported (e.g., performing forced labor in Nazi captivity), but too infrequently to be included in the Biographical Interview.

In addition, the 147 veterans only were interviewed using (a) the Clinical Rating Interview based on the original DSM-III (1980) criteria for PTSD [17]; and (b) the Structured Clinical Interview for PTSD as defined by DSM-III-R (1987) [18]. They also completed a questionnaire about their current health status [2].

The differences between veterans and heart and surgical patients were analyzed by means of χ^2 tests, t tests, and ANOVAs. All subjects were classified as suffering from 'vital exhaustion' if their score on the Maastricht Questionnaire was > 8.0. This cutoff point was the median score of both control groups combined used in the previous study [12, 13].

Results

Table 1 shows that the Resistance veterans, heart patients, and surgical patients differed significantly with respect to angina pectoris, smoking, type A behavior, 'vital exhaustion', and life stressors over the entire life-span, as included in the Biographical Interview. With the exception of smoking, the veterans had the highest scores. When the veterans were compared to heart patients of about the same age, they were more often assessed as type As ($p < 0.01$) and reported more 'vital exhaustion' ($p < 0.01$). They did not differ with respect to angina pectoris and life stressors, as assessed by the Biographical Interview, and they smoked less often ($p < 0.01$). When compared to surgical patients, veterans scored higher on all these risk factors except smoking. The remaining analyses will focus on CVD risk factors and current

Table 2. Clinical symptoms of current PTSD in WW II Resistance veterans according to the Clinical Rating Interview (DSM-III)

Symptoms	PTSD, % (n = 74)	No-PTSD, % (n = 62)
Intrusive recollections	90	22
Intensification of emotions	90	55
Sleep disturbances	87	44
Hyperalertness	73	38
Memory impairment	67	30
Avoidance of trauma resembling stimuli	67	41
Recurrent dreams	66	22
Constricted affect	63	13
Guilt feelings	63	27
Sudden acting as if trauma reoccurred	60	11
Feelings of detachment	57	11
Diminished interest	49	6

PTSD in Resistance veterans since PTSD was not studied in the heart and surgical patients.

According to the Structured Clinical Interview (1987) [18], 56% of *all* veterans were *currently* suffering from PTSD; this also occurred with 54% of the 74 veterans who underwent imprisonment in concentration camps. Therefore, participation in Resistance activities itself and living with the perpetual fear of being betrayed, imprisoned, and brought to death may have been more responsible for bringing about PTSD than the hardships of subsequent imprisonment itself. Table 2 shows that all 12 clinical PTSD symptoms, as assessed by means of the Clinical Rating Interview (1980) [17], were highly prevalent in veterans with current PTSD. Since these Rating Interviews could not be completed with all veterans, these data apply to 136 veterans only. The associations of current PTSD with anxiety, anger, and depression are reported elsewhere in this volume [17].

Table 3 shows that veterans with current PTSD, as assessed by means of the Structured Clinical Interview (1987) [18], and those without the disorder did not differ with respect to hypertension; about one third of *all* veterans indicated this. Furthermore, some 10% of *all* veterans reported having suffered an MI at least once within the past 15 years. With respect to angina pectoris and the CVD risk factors smoking, type A behavior, 'vital exhaustion', and life stressors, veterans with current PTSD scored highest. Because eight items assessing 'vital exhaustion' correspond to some criteria for current PTSD (in particular DSM-III-R categories C and D) and may thus constitute confounders, these items were omitted from further analysis. Yet, 'vital exhaustion' in veterans with current PTSD remained higher than in those without the disorder. Thus, the occurrence of 'vital exhaustion' in the former veterans was not confounded by these associations with current PTSD.

Of the 82 veterans with current PTSD, 67 (82%) were type As, as opposed to 41 (63%) of the 65 veterans without PTSD ($p < 0.05$). Moreover, type A veterans reported 'vital exhaustion' to a larger degree than type Bs ($p < 0.01$).

Life stressors, as included in the Biographical Interview, may also have confounded the prevalence of current PTSD since veterans with the disorder reported more such events.

Table 3. Cardiovascular disease risk factors in WW II Resistance veterans with current PTSD and in those without

Variables	PTSD (n = 82)	No-PTSD (n = 65)	p
Mean age	63.8	64.5	
SD	1.5	1.4	
Hypertension, %	32	31	NS
Angina pectoris, %	31	14	*
Prior MI, %	9	10	NS
Smoking, %	57	34	*
Type A behavior, %	82	63	*
Mean 'vital exhaustion'[1]	30.1	15.5	**
SD	9.9	10.9	
Mean 'vital exhaustion'[2]	19.4	9.6	**
SD	6.5	7.6	
Mean life stressors[3]	4.2	3.3	*
SD	2.1	1.5	

* p < 0.05; ** p < 0.001.
1 MQ 21 items.
2 MQ 13 items.
3 12 life stressors.

Therefore, these twelve stressors were analyzed separately. Prolonged financial problems (p < 0.01) and prolonged familial conflicts (p < 0.05) *prior* to WW II were more prevalent in the family life of veterans with current PTSD. *After* the war they encountered more prolonged marital conflicts (p < 0.001) and prolonged educational problems with children (p < 0.01) than veterans without the disorder. Life stressors associated with conflicts at work or their careers did not differ between the two groups.

Discussion

Fifty-six percent of these Dutch Resistance veterans from WW II, aged 60–65, were *currently* suffering from PTSD. Intrusive recollections and intensification of emotions were reported by almost all veterans suffering from the disorder. Sleep disturbances and hyperalertness were the most commonly reported behavioral symptoms. Since only a few studies have been conducted regarding the long-term health consequences of being a Resistance veteran, direct comparisons with other studies could not be made.

The observed current PTSD rate may be considered high. The prevalence of PTSD in Vietnam veterans seeking medical treatment has been assessed as being 46%, the highest in three groups of combat veterans [4]. In the Vietnam Experience Study, about 15% of their veterans experienced combat-related PTSD at some time after military service [3, 5]. In the general US population, this is estimated to be about 1% [20].

Of the current CVD risk factors, hypertension in Resistance veterans was reported at about the same rate (31–32%) as in the Vietnam Experience Study [5] and was not associated with current PTSD. The prevalence of prior MI (9–10%) and angina pectoris, which was significantly higher in veterans suffering from current PTSD (31%) than in those not suffering from it (14%), was higher than that in other veteran samples [5, 6]. Thus, these data about angina pectoris and MI could be said to support the hypothesis that PTSD may be associated with *excess* CVD in Vietnam veterans as they grow older [7, 8].

When compared to heart patients, Resistance veterans were more often type As. They were also much more 'vitally exhausted' than these heart patients of about the same age who had recently survived their first MIs [12]. Moreover, veterans with current PTSD were more often type As and they reported more 'vital exhaustion' than those without the disorder. Thus, these data suggest that type A behavior as a stable behavioral disposition over the life-span [21] may very well be associated with the occurrence of PTSD in subjects exposed to extreme war-time trauma and that, in conjunction, these may lead to severe manifestations of 'vital exhaustion'. Because the design of the present study was cross-sectional, this model could, however, not be tested.

Since current 'vital exhaustion' and PTSD have some aspects in common, in particular symptoms of avoidance and arousal, those possible confounders were omitted from analysis. Yet, veterans with current PTSD were found to suffer from 'vital exhaustion' to a more severe extent than those without the disorder. Thus, exposure to war-time trauma may be associated with severe current 'vital exhaustion'. This exhaustion reflects a state of 'excess fatigue' [10, 11, 13], which is not included in DSM-III-R defined PTSD.

The finding that veterans suffering from current PTSD differed from those not suffering from it with respect to two *prewar* life stressors, namely prolonged financial problems and prolonged familial conflicts (both in childhood and/or adolescence), deserves attention. These data suggest that premorbid adverse living conditions may have contributed to one's becoming more vulnerable to traumatic events. The scarce available evidence suggests that unfavorable conditions for family socialization during childhood and adolescence, such as represented by the present stressors, may sensitize subjects' attention to environmental cues that indicate threat [15]. Other studies indicate that adverse living conditions in childhood are associated with excess risk for CVD later in life [22, 23]. Thus, it may be hypothesized that the hyperalertness that was found in a large majority of the veterans with current PTSD, as well as the current prevalence rates of CVD risk factors, are associated with early sensitization to environmental stressors.

The present findings should, however, be considered with caution. This cross-sectional study was performed without a properly selected control group, and the information about the CVD risk factors was only obtained recently. Therefore, it would not be correct to calculate the estimated relative risks and confidence intervals for current PTSD associated with the present CVD risk factors since it would be impossible to determine whether those factors actually preceded current PTSD or whether they were a consequence of this disorder [24].

One may further wonder whether the present findings were influenced by selection bias, retrospective bias, or by confounding personality characteristics like 'neuroticism' in the participating Resistance veterans. Differences between participating and nonparticipating veterans with respect to mean scores on the questionnaires that would indicate selection bias could not be studied due to the latter's refusal to complete them. However, their reported reasons for nonparticipation were that they felt too old, too ill, too depressed, and above all, too exhausted to participate. Thus, selection bias may have influenced these findings to some extent. Yet, it may be argued that the participating veterans most likely represent the 'healthier' subjects from this age group.

Retrospective bias, due to sensitization to recent stress or trauma that they think may have contributed to their present state, may have led veterans with current PTSD to report more 'vital exhaustion' and cardiovascular complaints than they actually experienced. The substantial significant differences with respect to 'vital exhaustion' (also after omitting PTSD-related items), smoking, and angina pectoris that remain when veterans with current PTSD were compared with veterans without the disorder render this unlikely. Having become sensitized to recent stress or trauma appears, in itself, not enough reason to account for these elevated scores. Furthermore, it seems unlikely that this may lead to a higher prevalence of type A behavior among veterans with current PTSD since this is a stable behavioral disposition that, most probably, has characterized these veterans for decades. One may, therefore, conclude that the present findings are not influenced to a considerable extent by retrospective bias.

Finally, it could be argued that the higher prevalence of PTSD in general and of the CVD risk factors in particular in veterans with current PTSD does not represent their actual psychic or physical condition. Rather, 'neuroticism' as a common, basic psychometric component of many questionnaires about aspects of personal dysfunctioning, which represents a normally distributed personality characteristic, could also account for the present findings with respect to PTSD and 'vital exhaustion' [25]. Furthermore, in particular with respect to angina pectoris, 'neuroticism' may constitute a habitual tendency to report physical complaints in the absence of clinically manifest disease [26, 27]. Thus, 'neuroticism' may be positively associated with psychic and physical complaints but does not necessarily lead to disease, namely current PTSD and CVD. Since no measure of 'neuroticism' was included in the present study, this issue cannot be resolved here. The prevalence of current PTSD was not, however, assessed by means of self-reports but rather by using the standardized SCID interview procedure administered by experienced psychiatrists. Furthermore, it is unlikely that the substantial differences between veterans with current PTSD and those veterans without with respect to 'vital exhaustion' (on both versions of the MQ), were brought about by 'neuroticism' alone.

In sum, the objectively and impartially documented trauma during the Nazi occupation, to which these surviving Dutch Resistance veterans were exposed, are associated with high prevalence rates of current PTSD and risk factors for CVD and with 'vital exhaustion'. This latter state best describes the psychic and physical condition of these surviving veterans who are now entering 'old age'.

Acknowledgments

This is a revised version of a paper presented at the Symposium 'Co-Morbidity of Traumatic Stress Reactions'. This research was supported, in part, by grants from 'Stichting 1940–1945', Amsterdam, the Netherlands.

We would like to thank Mrs. Pamela Falger-Cohen, MA, for her editorial assistance.

References

1 Warmbrunn W: The Dutch under German Occupation. 1940–1945. Stanford, Stanford University Press, 1963.

2 Op den Velde W, Falger P, Hovens J, et al: Post traumatic stress disorder in Dutch Resistance veterans from World War II; in Wilson J, Rafael B (eds): International Handbook of Traumatic Stress Syndromes. New York, Plenum Press, in press.

3 The Centers for Disease Control Vietnam Experience Study: Health status of Vietnam veterans. I. Psychosocial characteristics. JAMA 1988;259:2701–2707.

4 Blake D, Keane T, Wine P, et al: Prevalence of PTSD symptoms in combat veterans seeking medical treatment. J Trauma Stress 1990;3:15–27.

5 The Centers for Disease Control Vietnam Experience Study: Health status of Vietnam veterans. II. Physical health. JAMA 1988;259:2708–2714.

6 Shalev A, Bleich A, Ursano R: Posttraumatic stress disorder: Somatic comorbidity and effort tolerance. Psychosomatics 1990;31:197–203.

7 Rosen J, Fields R: The long-term effects of extraordinary trauma: A look beyond PTSD. J Anxiety Disord 1988;2:179–191.
8 Blanchard E: Elevated basal levels of cardiovascular responses in Vietnam veterans with PTSD: A health problem in the making? J Anxiety Disord 1990;4:233–237.
9 Op den Velde W, Falger P, De Groen JHM, et al: Current psychiatric complaints of Dutch Resistance veterans from World War II: A feasibility study. J Trauma Stress, 1990;3:351–358.
10 Appels A: Mental precursors of myocardial infarction. Br J Psychiatry 1990;156:465–471.
11 Appels A, Mulder P: Excess fatigue as a precursor of myocardial infarction. Eur Heart J 1988;9:758–764.
12 Falger P, Schouten E, Appels A, et al: Sleep complaints, behavioral characteristics and vital exhaustion in myocardial infarction cases. Psychol Health 1988;2:231–258.
13 Falger P: Life-span development and myocardial infarction: An epidemiological study; PhD thesis, University of Limburg School of Medicine, Maastricht, 1989.
14 Appels A, Schouten E: Waking up exhausted as risk indicator of myocardial infarction. Am J Cardiol 1991;68:395–398.
15 Compas B: Coping with stress during childhood and adolescence. Psychol Bull 1987;101:393–403.
16 Rosenman R: The interview method of assessment of the coronary-prone behavior pattern; in Dembroski T, Weiss S, Shields J, et al (eds): Coronary-Prone Behavior. New York, Springer, 1978.
17 American Psychiatric Association: Diagnostic and statistical manual of mental disorders. 3rd ed. Washington, American Psychiatric Press, 1980.
18 American Psychiatric Association: Diagnostic and statistical manual of mental disorders, 3rd rev ed. Washington, American Psychiatric Press, 1987.
19 Hovens J, Op den Velde W, Falger P, et al: Anxiety, depression, and anger in Dutch Resistance veterans from World War II. Psychother Psychosom 1992;57:172–179.
20 Helzer J, Robins L, McEvoy L: Posttraumatic stress disorder in the general population. N Engl J Med 1987; 317:1630–1634.
21 Matthews K, Haynes S: Type A behavior pattern and coronary disease risk: Update and critical evaluation. Am J Epidemiol 1986;123:923–960.
22 Forsdahl A: Living conditions in childhood and subsequent development of risk factors for arteriosclerotic heart disease. J Epidemiol Community Health 1978;32:34–47.
23 Arnesen E, Forsdahl A: The Tromso heart study: Coronary risk factors and their association with living conditions during childhood. J Epidemiol Community Health 1985; 39:210–214.
24 Rothman K: Modern Epidemiology. Boston, Little, Brown, 1986.
25 Luteijn F, Bouman T: The concepts of depression, anxiety, and neuroticism in questionnaires. Eur J Pers 1988;2:113–120.
26 Costa P Jr, Zonderman A, Engel B, et al: The relation of chest pain symptoms to angiographic findings of coronary artery stenosis and neuroticism. Psychosom Med 1985;47: 285–293.
27 Costa P Jr: Influence of the normal personality dimension of neuroticism on chest pain symptoms and coronary heart disease. Am J Cardiol 1987;60:20J–26J.

2nd Europ Conf on Traumatic Stress
Psychother Psychosom 1992;57:172–179

Johannes E. Hovens[a, b]
Wybrand Op den Velde[b]
Paul R.J. Falger[c]
Eric G.W. Schouten[c]
Johannes H.M. De Groen[d]
Hans Van Duijn[e]

[a] Centrum 45, National Center for the Treatment of WW II Victims, Oegstgeest;
[b] Department of Psychiatry, St. Lucas Hospital, Amsterdam;
[c] Department of Medical Psychology;
[d] Department of Clinical Neurophysiology, University of Limburg School of Medicine, Maastricht;
[e] Department of Clinical Neurophysiology, St. Lucas Hospital, Amsterdam, The Netherlands

Anxiety, Depression and Anger in Dutch Resistance Veterans from World War II

Key Words
Posttraumatic stress disorder
World War II
Resistance veterans
Anxiety
Depresssion
Anger

Abstract
In this study, 147 Dutch Resistance veterans from WW II are evaluated on psychometric instruments for anxiety, depression and anger. Resistance veterans appeared to be more anxious, depressive and angry on these instruments compared to controls from the validation studies of the respective instruments. Veterans currently suffering from PTSD (56%) were significantly more anxious, depressed, and angry than veterans without PTSD. With respect to staying in Nazi concentration camps, which is an extremely severe stressor, and in which half of the veterans were imprisoned, no difference on the three instruments was found. Anxiety, depression and anger were observed to be highly interrelated in PTSD. The close interrelationship between anxiety and depression, anxiety and danger, and depression and anger mediated by way of anxiety is, however, not unique for traumatized subjects. It is argued that for Resistance veterans only the intrusive reminiscences of the stressful events discriminate this constellation of symptoms from subjects with an anxious-depressive symptomatology.

Introduction

DSM-III-R [1] defines posttraumatic stress disorder (PTSD) as an anxiety disorder. While in the current notion of PTSD intrusive reminiscences of the constituent event are a necessary condition to diagnose the disorder [2] in earlier publications both anxiety symptoms (e.g. nervousness, restlessness, irritability, phobias, and chronic anxiety) and depres-

J.E. Hovens
Centrum 45
Rijnzichtweg 35
NL–2342 AX Oegstgeest (The Netherlands)

sive symptoms (e.g. apathy, withdrawal, sleep disturbances, and guilt feelings), formed the core of PTSD [3]. Futterman and Pumpian-Mindlin [4] were probably the first to characterize 'intense anxiety' as primary symptoms in traumatic war neurosis, and 'a tendency to avoid people' as secondary symptoms. Chronic anxiety neurosis and chronic depressive reactions in concentration camp survivors were described in 1968 [5]. Psychometric support for anxiety and depressive symptoms in PTSD was reported by Fairbank et al. [6] on 36 Vietnam veterans. Twelve veterans with PTSD had significantly elevated scores on the Zung depression scale and on the Spielberger State-Trait Anxiety Inventory, compared to combat veterans without PTSD and noncombat psychiatric inpatients. Comparable findings with the Beck Depression Inventory and the State Trait Anxiety Inventory are described by Orr et al. [7], who contrasted 25 Vietnam combat veterans, suffering from PTSD, with 7 anxious and 18 healthy combat veterans.

The association of depression and war experiences is suggested by Helzer et al. [8]. They found a 7% prevalence rate for full major affective disorder in their random sample of 470 Vietnam veterans, and some symptoms of depression in 26%. While Nace et al. [9] reported that in their sample of 202 Vietnam veterans, who were either hospitalized or in a drug treatment program, 33% fell within the clinically depressed range of the Beck Depression Inventory, the Helzer et al. [10] follow-up study did not find a higher incidence of depression in their combat veterans 3 years after returning to the United States compared to the matched civilian controls. This may indicate that depressive symptoms fade with time. On the other hand, in an Australian study it was shown that a random sample of 170 prisoners of war (POW) from World War II (WW II) was significantly more depressed on the Zung depression scale than matched veterans without POW experience 40 years after the POW experience [11]. This study suggests that the severely stressful event of a Japanese POW camp may have an impact on depression, even after 40 years. It should, however, be noted that none of these studies related the depressive symptomatology to PTSD.

As far as anxiety symptoms are concerned, MMPI-based data in 41 former WW II POWs, half of them suffering from current PTSD, suggest a profound anxiety state with depressive features [12], which matches the clinical impression about anxiety symptoms in former POWs and concentration camp survivors. Tennant et al. [13] did not find any significant statistical differences on trait anxiety in 170 randomly selected POWs from WW II compared to veterans with no POW experience. These contradictory findings may imply that comparing POWs with highly stressed war veterans on psychometric instruments for anxiety is not suitable. This is supported by the finding that these POWs had a greater risk for any clinical psychiatric diagnosis, clinical anxiety disorder and clinical depressive disorder other than major depression, while the latter almost reached significance compared to veterans without POW experience [14]. In these studies the relationship between PTSD and anxiety was not investigated.

As anxiety and depression appear to be related to war stressors and to PTSD, another approach to illuminate this relationship is to examine whether specific war stressors predict clinical diagnoses other than PTSD [15, 16]. In 69 hospitalized Vietnam veterans, 77% suffering from PTSD, participation in atrocities and number of combat stressors appeared to predict PTSD, and to a much lesser extent panic disorder [15]. In the Green et al. [16] study with 200 help-seeking and nonhelp-seeking Vietnam veterans, 29% of the veterans fulfilled the criteria for PTSD, while PTSD as the only diagnosis was present in 3.6% of the sample. War time stressors appeared to predict best PTSD in combination with panic disorder.

In sum, the associations of anxiety and depression with PTSD may be thought to be complex. First of all, the relation between a specific war stressor on the one hand and anxiety and depression on the other hand might be involved. Secondly, it might be thought that the war stress in general does differentiate the veterans from civilian controls. Thirdly, anxiety and depression may go hand in hand with PTSD. It should be noted that a cooccurrence of depressive mood disorder is reported in 33% of psychiatric patients having an anxiety disorder [17], and psychometric correlations between anxiety and depression range from 0.60 to 0.73 [18].

Apart from anxiety and depression, anger might also be involved. To our knowledge anger has not yet been studied in connection with PTSD. The clinical impression is, however, that most of the veterans feel aggressive towards and abandoned by society and authorities. The interrelationships between anxiety, depression, and anger in relationship to PTSD needs further exploration.

The purpose of the present study is, therefore (1) to compare Dutch Resistance veterans from WW II with validated data from the population with respect to anxiety, depression and anger. It is expected that veterans have higher scores on all three measures; (2) to compare PTSD subjects with non-PTSD subjects. It is hypothesized that PTSD subjects have higher scores on all three measures; (3) to compare PTSD subjects with non-PTSD subjects with respect to a specific war stressor, i.e. captivity in a Nazi concentration camp. It is hypothesized that PTSD subjects with concentrations camp experience have higher scores on all three measures, and (4) to explore the interrelations between anxiety, depression and anger.

Method

Subjects. As a formal registration of Dutch WW II Resistance veterans never took place, all of those male veterans between 60 and 65 years of age as of January 1, 1986, registered with the Dutch 'Stichting 1940–1945' and living in the Netherlands (n = 813), were asked to participate. The 'Stichting 1940–1945' is a government-supported, private foundation that actively promotes the general interests of former Dutch Resistance veterans and their next-of-kin. The foundation is responsible for investigating and acknowledging the factual Resistance records of all veterans applying for an extraordinary government-financed veterans' disability pension. In each case, this is done by means of a series of impartial witnesses' reports. In this manner, the objectively documented Resistance history of each veteran has been made accessible for research. Of all the initially contacted subjects, 619 (76%) agreed to participate in the study. From these veterans a sample of 182 subjects was drawn. Complete questionnaires and interview data were collected from 147 subjects (81%). More details about the selection procedure and the instruments are described elsewhere [19, 20].

Instruments. The following self-report measures were included: (1) The Spielberger Trait-Anxiety Inventory [20] in the Dutch adaptation [21, 22]. This scale measures individual differences in the disposition to experience anxiety and consists of 20 items; (2) the Spielberger Trait-Anger scale [23] in the Dutch adaptation [24]. This scale consists of 10 items and measures individual differences in the disposition to experience anger, and (3) the Zung Self-Rating Depression scale [25] in the Dutch adaptation [26–28], consisting of 20 items, and measuring individual differences in the disposition to experience depression. On the instruments above, evidence on reliability and validity is widely available [21, 22, 24, 27, 28]; (4) furthermore, an interview session at home included a rating of the presence of current PTSD by means of the Structured Clinical Interview (SCID) for DSM-II-R defined PTSD [29].

Procedure. All subjects (n = 813) were sent a letter requesting their participation in a study on psychic and physical determinants of current sleep disturbances in Resistance veterans. The sample of 182 veterans was sent an additional set of psychological

Table 1. Mean scores for anxiety, depression and anger scales in Resistance veterans

	All[1] veterans	PTSD[2]	Non-PTSD[3]	Population
Anxiety score	47.95	54.00	39.35	38.2[4]
SD	12.66	9.98	11.03	11.7
n	126	74	52	60
Depression score	45.71	50.59	38.83	35.2[5]
SD	10.59	8.16	9.83	6.8
n	128	75	53	92
Anger score	20.67	22.41	18.19	17.4[6]
SD	6.72	7.28	4.92	5.9
n	126	74	52	60

1 t tests between all veterans and population controls: $p < 0.001$ for anxiety, and depression. $p = 0.001$ for anger.
2 t tests between PTSD subjects and non-PTSD subjects: $p < 0.001$ for anxiety, depression, and anger.
3 t tests between non-PTSD subjects and population controls: p = non-significant for anxiety, and anger. $p = 0.005$ for depression.
4 Van der Ploeg [22].
5 Mook et al. [27, 28].
6 Van der Ploeg et al. [24].

and health questionnaires. The 147 subjects (81%) who returned this set of questionnaires were subsequently interviewed at home. Some questionnaires were completed only partially (i.e. 2 items or more missing), and were not used for further statistical analyses. This applied to 21 anxiety, 21 anger, and 19 depression questionnaires, respectively.

Results

According to the SCID ratings, 82 veterans (56%) were identified as currently suffering from PTSD, whereas 65 (44%) were not. The total number of subjects for the three instruments varies between 126 and 128 due to incomplete questionnaires. Means and standard deviations on the anxiety, anger and depression scales were computed for the total sample of Resistance veterans, as well as for the subgroups, PTSD and non-PTSD subjects, according to the SCID. The results are presented in table 1. It shows that the mean scores are significantly higher in Resistance veterans from WW II compared to older males (i.e. > 40 years) in the population from the Dutch validation studies of the respective instruments. For anxiety $t = 5.0$ (d.f. 184; $p < 0.001$); for depression $t = 7.0$ (d.f. = 186; $p < 0.001$), and for anger $t = 3.21$ (d.f. = 184; $p = 0.001$). These results are consistent with the hypothesis that Resistance veterans are more anxious, depressed and angry than civilian controls. However, it should be noted that the subjects in the present study are substantially older, as their age range was limited from 60 to 65 years, while in the validation studies age ranged from 41 to 70 years.

The comparison of the non-PTSD subjects with the validation controls showed that non-PTSD subjects did not differ on the anxiety and anger measures from the controls. On the depression measure non-PTSD subjects had a

Table 2. Trait intercorrelations for anxiety, depression and anger in PTSD and non-PTSD Resistance veterans

Subjects	n	Scales	Anger	Depression
All	124	1 anxiety	0.58 (0.38)	0.88 (0.85)
		2 anger		0.48 (–0.08)
PTSD	73	1 anxiety	0.48 (0.39)	0.80 (0.77)
		2 anger		0.33 (–0.09)
Non-PTSD	51	1 anxiety	0.64 (0.40)	0.84 (0.77)
		2 anger		0.55 (0.02)

higher score than the controls ($t = 2.60$; $p = 0.005$). The differences between Resistance veterans and controls on anxiety and anger, then, may be attributed to the scores of the PTSD subjects. The comparison of PTSD subjects with non-PTSD subjects showed that PTSD subjects had higher scores on all three measures, suggesting that subjects suffering from PTSD are more anxious, depressed and angry, which corresponds with the hypothesis. For all three t tests $p < 0.001$, with $t = -7.77$ (d.f. = 124) for anxiety, $t = -7.36$ (d.f. = 126) for depression and $t = -3.63$ (d.f. = 124) for anger.

Seventy-four Resistance veterans were imprisoned in concentration camps, subsequent to their Resistance work, and 41 of them (55%) currently suffered from PTSD. Since an equal number of the 73 veterans, who had not been imprisoned in concentration camps, also suffered from current PTSD (n = 41, 56%), there was no difference between both subgroups with respect to the occurrence of PTSD (χ^2 = nonsignificant). No significant relation could be demonstrated for anxiety, depression or anger and PTSD, with the specific war stressor 'concentration camp imprisonment' as an intervening variable ($F = 0.23$; $p = 0.64$, $F = 0.07$; $p = 0.80$, and $F = 3.1$; $p = 0.08$ for anxiety, depression, and anger, respectively), thus refuting the hypothesis. The intercorrelations between anxiety, depression and anger were computed for all Resistance veterans, and for PTSD and for non-PTSD subjects. The first-order partial correlation coefficients were computed in order to control statistically for the effects of each measure on the relationship between the others. The results are presented in table 2, with the partial correlations in parentheses. Table 2 shows that the correlations for all three measures are statistically significant beyond the 0.01 level for the total sample, as well as for both subgroups. The correlation between anxiety and depression appears to be strongest, suggesting that both instruments have much in common in Resistance veterans. The correlation between anxiety and anger is less strong, while for anger and depression the correlation is the lowest, though still substantial. The partial correlations show that the correlations between anxiety and depression, and between anxiety and anger are not substantially affected. For the relationship between anger and depression, however, the correlations are no longer significant. This suggests that the positive correlation for anger and depression in the total sample, and in the two subgroups, is mediated by anxiety.

Discussion

Studies relating current symptomatology of anxiety, anger, depression and PTSD to WW II and Vietnam war stressors are not easy to compare. One study with random community sampling among subjects who served in Vietnam compared depressive symptoms of these subjects with symptoms in civilian controls [10]. This study, however, did not control for specific PTSD symptomatology. Another aspect is that adjustment problems after severely stressful events might first present itself as anxiety symptoms, which change to depressive features with elapsing time [30]. In other studies subjects with POW experience were compared to combat veterans [11, 13], or subjects were evaluated with regard to specific war stressors [15, 16]. These studies might underestimate the occurrence of anxiety and depression, as all subjects underwent severe stressors, although the relative effect of several stressors can be evaluated. Finally, in some studies PTSD subjects are compared with non-PTSD subjects and nonveterans [6, 7]. These studies are, however, very limited in the number of subjects, and could not discriminate between a variety of stressors.

In our investigation we were able to compare 147 Resistance veterans, whose stressful experiences in WW II are impartially documented, with the data of the validation studies for the three used instruments. Clearly, Resistance veterans showed, more than 40 years after the war, more symptoms of anxiety, depression and anger than the controls from the validation studies. As non-PTSD subjects did not differ on anxiety and anger from the controls, these differences for the Resistance veterans, as a group, may be explained by the scores of the PTSD subjects. The subjects with current PTSD appeared to have significantly higher scores than the non-PTSD veterans. These results are consistent with the findings from the studies which compared PTSD subjects with non-PTSD subjects and nonveterans [6, 7]. They also show that symptoms do not completely wane with time. This is also reflected in the higher depression score of the non-PTSD subjects compared to the controls. Depression has been suggested to form the end stage of PTSD [20]. On the other hand, PTSD is not a static disorder but may have its remissions and exacerbations [19]. Thus, when anxiety, depression and anger scores are significantly higher in PTSD veterans, this suggests that anxiety, depression and anger are embedded in PTSD.

Half of the Resistance veterans were imprisoned in concentration camps. Although the Nazi concentration camps, in particular the annihilation camps, can probably be considered as one of the most severe stressors conceivable, the results showed no influence of this specific stressor on PTSD and on the anxiety, depression and anger measures. This means that continuous stress, such as Resistance veterans without concentration camp imprisonment underwent, cannot be simply differentiated from the stress to which Resistance veterans with these imprisonments experiences were submitted. It might be possible that concentration camp victims have more periods of PTSD, which our data do not show, but which is suggested by the findings from a study by Tennant et al. [14]. It might also be possible that in concentration camp survivors symptoms other than anxiety, depression or anger are important, thus reflecting differences in the severity of the stressor. As far as current anxiety, depression and anger on psychometric instruments are concerned, however, no difference appeared.

How are anxiety, depression and anger related to each other? All three measures appeared to be highly related to each other, while the first-order partial correlations showed that the relation between anger and depression was mediated by anxiety. An interpretation of these results is that uncontrollable anxiety makes one angry, while continuous anxiety leads to exhaustion, manifesting itself in depressive symptoms. This interpretation is consistent with earlier descriptions of the PTSD syndrome. However, findings in other populations show similar relations between these three concepts [18]. This means that the constellation of anxiety, depression and anger in Resistance veterans from WW II does not form a unique constellation of symptoms. An anxious-depressive complex of symptoms is common in subjects suffering from anxiety disorders [17]. This suggests that the uniqueness of PTSD in Resistance veterans, and probably in all traumatized subjects, lies in the nature of the stressful events and the intrusive reminiscences of these events.

Acknowledgement

This study was supported, in part, by grant No. 83.002 from 'Stichting Dienstverlening Verzetsdeelnemers', Dirkshorn, the Netherlands, and by grant No. 84.012 from 'Stichting 1940–1945', Amsterdam, The Netherlands.

References

1 American Psychiatric Association: Diagnostic and Statistical Manual of Mental Disorders, ed 3 revised. Washington, APA, 1987.

2 Brett EA, Spitzer RL, Williams JBW: DSM-III-R criteria for posttraumatic stress disorder. Am J Psychiatry 1988;145:1232–1236.

3 Ettedgui E, Bridges M: Posttraumatic stress disorder. Psychiatr Clin North Am 1985;8:89–103.

4 Futterman S, Pumpian-Mindlin E: Traumatic war neuroses five years later. Am J Psychiatry 1951;108:401–408.

5 Häfner H: Psychological disturbances following prolonged persecution. Soc Psychiatry 1968;3:79–88.

6 Fairbank JA, Keane TM, Malloy PF: Some preliminary data on the psychological characteristics of Vietnam veterans with Posttraumatic Stress Disorders. J Consult Clin Psychol 1983;51:912–919.

7 Orr SP, Claiborn JM, Altman B, Forgue DF, De Jong JB, Pitman RK, Herz LR: Psychometric profile of Posttraumatic Stress Disorder, anxious, and healthy Vietnam Veterans: Correlations with psychophysiologic responses. J Consult Clin Psychol 1990;58:329–335.

8 Helzer JE, Robins LN, Davis DH: Depressive disorders in Vietnam returnees. J Nerv Ment Dis 1976;163:177–185.

9 Nace EP, Meyers AL, O'Brien CP, Ream N, Mintz J: Depression in veterans two years after Vietnam. Am J Psychiatry 1977;134:167–170.

10 Helzer JE, Robins LN, Wish E, Hesselbrock M: Depression in Vietnam veterans and civilian controls. Am J Psychiatry 1979;136:526–529.

11 Dent OF, Tennant CC, Goulston KJ: Precursors of depression in world war II veterans 40 years after the war. J Nerv Ment Dis 1987;175:486–490.

12 Goldstein G, van Kammen W, Shelly C, Miller DJ, Van Kammen DP: Survivors of imprisonment in the Pacific theater during world war II. Am J Psychiatry 1987;144:1210–1213.

13 Tennant CC, Goulston KJ, Dent OF: The psychological effects of being a prisoner-of-war: Forty years after release. Am J Psychiatry 1986;143:618–621.

14 Tennant CC, Goulston KJ, Dent OF: Clinical psychiatric illness in prisoners of war of the Japanese: Forty years after release. Psychol Med 1986;16:833–839.

15 Breslau N, Davis GC: Posttraumatic stress disorder: the etiologic specificity of wartime stressors. Am J Psychiatry 1987;144:578–583.

16 Green BL, Lindy JD, Grace MC, Gleser GC: Multiple diagnosis in Posttraumatic Stress Disorder: The role of war stressors. J Nerv Ment Dis 1989;177:329–335.

17 Sanderson WC, DiNardo PA, Rapee RM, Barlow DH: Syndrome comorbidity in patients diagnosed with a DSM-III-R Anxiety Disorder. J Abnorm Psychol 1990;99:308–312.

18 Mook J, Van der Ploeg HM, Kleijn WChr: anxiety, anger and depression: Relationships at the trait level. Anxiety Res 1990;3:17–31.

19 Op den Velde W, Falger PRJ, Hovens JE, De Groen JHM, Lasschuit LJ, Van Duijn H, Schouten EGW: PTSD in Dutch Resistance veterans from World War II; in Wilson JP, Rafael B (eds): The International Handbook of Traumatic Stress Syndromes. New York, Plenum Press, 1992.

20 Falger PRJ, Op den Velde W, Hovens JE, Schouten EGW, De Groen JHM, Van Duyn H: Current Posttraumatic Stress Disorder and cardiovascular disease risk factors in Dutch Resistance veterans from WW II. Psychother Psychosom 1992;57:164–171.

20 Spielberger CD: Manual for the State-Trait Anxiety Inventory STAI-form Y. Palo Alto, Consulting Psychologists Press, 1983.

21 Ploeg HM van der, Defares PB, Spielberger CD: Handleiding bij de Zelf-Beoordelings Vragenlijst, ZBV. Lisse, Swets & Zeitlinger, 1980.
22 Ploeg HM van der: Zelf-Beoordelings Vragenlijst Addendum. Lisse, Swets & Zeitlinger, 1981.
23 Spielberger CD, Jacobs G, Russell S, Crane RS: Assessment of anger: The State-Trait Anger Scale; in Butcher JN, Spielberger CD (eds): Advances in Personality Assessment. Hillsdale, Erlbaum, 1983, vol 2, pp 159–187.
24 Ploeg HM van der, Defares PB, Spielberger CD: Handleiding bij de Zelfanalyse Vragenlijst (ZAV). Lisse, Swets & Zeitlinger, 1982.
25 Zung WWK: A Self-Rating Depression Scale. Arch Gen Psychiatry 1965;12:63–70.
26 Dijkstra P: De Zelfbeoordelingsschaal voor depressie van Zung; in Van Praag HM, Rooijmans HGM (eds): Stemming en Ontstemming: Theorie en praktijk bij de diagnostiek en behandeling van depressie. Amsterdam, De Erven Bohn, 1974.
27 Mook J, Kleijn WChr, Van der Ploeg HM: Een herziene Nederlandse versie van de Zung-schaal als maat voor dispositionele depressiviteit. Tijdschr Psychiat 1989;32:253–264.
28 Mook J, Kleijn WChr, Van der Ploeg HM: Depressiviteit als dispositie gemeten met de Zung-schaal: Interne structuur en relaties met angst, boosheid, coping en sociale steun. Ned Tijdschr Psychol 1989; 44:328–340.
29 Spitzer RL, Williams JBW, Gibbon M: Instruction manual for the Structured Clinical Interview for DSM-III-R. New York, Bio-metrics Research Department, 1985.
30 Lindy JD, Titchener J: 'Acts of God and man': Long-term character change in survivors of disasters and the law. Behav Sci Law 1983;1:85–96.

2nd Europ Conf on Traumatic Stress
Psychother Psychosom 1992;57:180–186

Jacob D. Lindy
Bonnie L. Green
Mary Grace

University of Cincinnati
Traumatic Stress Study Center,
Cincinnati, Ohio, USA

Somatic Reenactment in the Treatment of Posttraumatic Stress Disorder

Key Words
Somatic reenactment
PTSD
Dynamic psychotherapy
Conversion reaction
Working alliance
Somatic symptoms in PTSD

Abstract
Somatic reenactments, like other intrusive symptoms in posttraumatic stress disorder, such as flashbacks and nightmares, reproduce the mental content of traumatic events. Four cases are presented from survivors of military trauma and civilian catastrophes. The patients were part of larger research projects carried out by the University of Cincinnati Traumatic Stress Study Center. Understanding such symptoms as repetitions of the trauma itself proved useful therapeutically, especially in consolidating the working alliance.

Somatic symptoms are often described in patients with posttraumatic stress disorder (PTSD) and in fact may be among the more pressing presenting clinical problems. The differential diagnosis of coexisting somatic states with PTSD may be complex, and treatment will of course vary with the etiology in the specific case. While contemporary PTSD literature appropriately emphasizes a physiologic component to trauma, especially autonomic hyperarousal, it is important to include in our differential diagnosis those somatic features which may be of psychogenic origin. Of special interest for this paper is one form of psychogenic somatic symptom in PTSD: *somatic reenactment.* This is a repetitive set of physical symptoms which is atypical in its composition from familiar pathophysiologic conditions. The symptoms themselves contain a somatic repetition of the trauma itself. It functions like other intrusive phenomena such as flashbacks and nightmares. The decoding of the somatic reenactment into the memory of the trauma patient becomes a central component in the different phases of the dynamic psychotherapy of patients with PTSD. The current paper illustrates this phenomenon in different posttrauma samples

Jacob D. Lindy, MD
3001 Highland Avenue
Cincinnati, OH 45219-2315 (USA)

0033–3190/92/
0574–0180$2.75/0

and identifies the role played by interpretation of the somatic reenactments in the treatments.

Somatic features have long been recognized as integral features in many posttrauma states [1–4]. By the midseventies, when an American task force took on the challenge of defining PTSD, Kadushin, et al. [5] reviewed the symptomatology of postwar syndromes in Western wars. They found that in over 75% of reported posttraumatic syndromes there were somatic components described. Most common were cardiopulmonary (asthma), central nervous system (headache and dizziness), and gastrointestinal (upset stomach, diarrhea). But neither DSM III nor DSM III-R contained a clearly demarcated area for somatic symptoms in PTSD except for those connected with the fright flight response itself. This decision apparently was because somatic disturbances, while often present, were not a sufficiently discriminating component in the disorder. The dearth of American research interest in somatic aspects of PTSD in the early 1980s may have been related.

Solomon and Mikuliner [6] and Solomon et al. [7], studying Israeli soldiers following combat in Lebanon, showed that veterans with PTSD, exhibit more somatic symptoms than those without PTSD both 1 year and 2 years after combat. But Shalev et al. [8] found that medical examination and laboratory studies at 5 years failed to distinguish the two groups. This discrepancy between somatic complaints and diagnosable medical illness holds for Vietnam veterans as well [9]. The authors appropriately emphasize the need for caution in interpretation of self-reports. But the extent to which reported symptoms differ from physical and biological findings may also define a domain of psychogenic symptom distress in PTSD.

In our work as clinicians and researchers at the University of Cincinnati Traumatic Stress Study Center we have similarly been impressed by the prominence of somatic features in the groups of survivors we have studied extensively: inhabitants of Buffalo Creek, West Virginia, whose valley was destroyed by a dam collapse and flood (125 dead) in 1972; patrons, rescue workers, employees, and next of kin survivors of supper club fire near Cincinnati, Ohio (165 dead) in 1977, and combat veterans of the Vietnam War.

Among survivors in our several studies who sought treatment, over one third described physical symptoms in their presenting complaints. These include a wide spectrum of somatic conditions and probable etiologies. Some were direct pathophysiological outcomes of the disaster as for example persistent cough as a result of chemical toxic bronchitis following exposure to fumes at the supper club fire, or complications of war injury among Vietnam veterans; some were traditional psychosomatic disorders as peptic ulcer disease. Some were preoccupation with vague aches, pains and fatigue as a somatitizing response to general anxiety especially in the rural Appalachian culture of Buffalo Creek in which somatization is more acceptable than 'mental condition'. Finally there were some survivors whose complaints appeared specific, recurrent, painful, yet atypcial and not easily explained on the basis of either physical etiology or (as it turned out) conventional conversion reaction. Some of these atypical somatic symptoms contained memories, in concrete form of the trauma itself. The pain of these physical symptoms reenacted traumatic affect in disassociated form. It is this latter phenomenon, somatic reenactment of trauma, and how it emerged and was dealt with within psychotherapy, which is the central focus of this paper.

Such work became an important part of the focal psychoanalytic treatment of patients in several of our studies [10]. The general design for the focal psychoanalytic treatment of PTSD, about which our group has written considerably, includes an opening phase in which the survivor chooses to trust the therapist in hope that sharing details of the trauma will lead to meaning or relief [10]. In the middle phase the therapist helps the patient identify the contours of the special configuration of the traumatic events; what triggers reminders of the event currently, and what coping responses this has set in place. In the final phase, the dyadic pair work on the meaning of the trauma experience to the person's self configuration and sense of continuity in time.

Among the troublesome traumatic intrusions of everyday life available to the therapist in each of these phases are somatic reenactments.

Case Reports

Case 1. Three months following a devastating supper club fire outside Cincinnati, Ohio, Mrs. F., a 48-year-old Black woman, presented for treatment. She had developed persistent urinary urgency without dysuria. The urgency was intense, forced her to excuse herself from routine activities and to go to the lavatory where she would usually pass a small amount of urine without much relief. A full-scale genitourinary work-up was negative. In the course of her psychological treatment, the patient recounted in detail her experiences at the fire. Mrs. F. had been a member of a gospel chorus which had been celebrating its annual outing the night of the fire. (The group was located in a special room on the second floor). When the lights went out, the group made a human chain and with utmost discipline and rather moving faith, they exited down a dark stairway, finding a safe exit. The entire group was safe, except for her two best friends. In psychotherapy Mrs. F. remembered that some moments before the lights went out these friends had asked her if she wanted to join them in the lavatory. Mrs. F., in retrospect, became aware of sensing her bladder, and finding that there was no urgency, she had said 'no' to her friends. They went off to the lavatory, the door became sealed during the fire and they were burned to death. Mrs. F.'s symptom repetitively captured the moment when she, sensing no pressure on her bladder, chose not to join her friends while they, sensing full bladders, went to their death. Discovering the symptom as traumatic reenactment ushered in a period of intense guilt, grief and mourning. She recalled many past events in her relationship with her friends, including negative ones; she confronted frustrations in her current life and wishes to join them in death. A dream that her friends were safe in heaven and were encouraging her to go on with her own life was reassuring, letting go of her symptom was like letting go of her unconscious attachment to them in death. Along with the remitting of the symptom, and the grieving for her friends, Mrs. F. reported a return to vigor in her current life.

Case 2. A pastor assisted families through a temporary morgue to identify their loved ones after the supper club fire. Six months later he sought help for pain in his left heel. The pain was extremely sharp 'as if to the bone' and was unremitting. He had a limp and had gone from one orthopedist to another in search of diagnosis and relief. Work-ups were all negative. As he recounted his experiences at the morgue he became aware of a previously forgotten detail. He was guiding a family through the morgue to identify their 17-year-old daughter. Hoping against hopes that she would not be there, the group actually passed the youngster without recognizing her. The priest however, checking the tag attached to the left heel of each of the cadavers read her name. It was he then who turned to the parents with the news that, what they wished so much not to be true, was indeed the case. The youngster before them was their daughter and she was dead. Rev. P. was exquisitely in tune with the painful loss this family experienced. He now recalled the death of his sister as a 17-year-old in an accident, and how close he had felt with her. The heel pain temporarily reestablished his painful connection with his dead sister as well as his absorbing the pain of this family.

For Mrs. F and Rev. P interpretation of somatic reenactment consolidated the working alliance. The psychogenic origin of the symptom was the therapist's key to entering beneath the survivor's trauma membrane and there unlock strong affect concerning death and trauma.

Case 3. Josh, a 35-year-old Appalachian man presented because of recurrent pain in his chest and abdomen. The symptom was rather striking and specific. It was extremely severe, like no other pain that he had endured previously. It was accompanied by a sensation of panic and imminent death. The pain appeared on the left side of the chest wall but initially the patient was unable to localize it more precisely. He responded compliantly to all medical questions about its radiation, etc. Characteristically, he would awaken at night with this 'heart' pain, be rushed to the hospital, where electrocardiographs would be performed and no abnormalities would be found. The patient did not connect the pain with any emotional stress.

Later, in psychotherapy, Josh explained that in Vietnam he had been passenger as a truck approached a small village at dusk where children were playing in the road. The driver, fearing the children might be carrying weapons, actually sped up as he got close to them and ran over a Vietnamese girl. Josh's therapiest considered several alternatives before settling on the chest pain as reenactment of trauma. Earlier explorations considered the symptom in light of nonspecific anxiety-related somatization. As the therapist was able to hear more clearly the specific nature of the symptoms described, he understood that the severe chest pain was indeed a rib sticking through a chest wall, the actual scene which the patient saw as he turned around and observed the little girl whom they had run over. The truck had crushed the child's chest. In retrospect, the children were most likely friendly to the Americans and he, the patient, felt enormous guilt.

Josh felt relieved by the interpretation of his somatic memory. He cried over the death of the child and with that grieving process opened up he discovered many connections to current inhibitions with his own children.

Case 4. Lee was a 36-year-old former combat Marine who experienced 2 years of heavy combat duty in Vietnam and Laos. Early in his treatment, the therapist noted that a particular physical symptom evolved often when the patient felt 'pinned down' or 'overrun' in civilian life, as for example, when his car was blocked in his driveway, or neighbors seemed to be harassing him. As he would describe these events, he would note a severe headache which on closer evaluation was rather unusual. It was circumscribed roughly circular, perhaps 10 cm in diameter, located in the left temporal area. During the conduct of this particular psychotherapy, the therapist was active in connecting physical sensations and emotional states of the present with unremembered events of Vietnam. In pursuing this actively the patient described the following scene: his unit was being overrun. There were VC all around, his bayonet was not affixed to his rifle and yet he had to use an instrument to protect himself in hand-to-hand combat. A Vietcong came up from his right side, the patient turned on him with the barrel of the rifle and crushed the skull of the enemy. He turned and saw a young boy and the crushed piece of skull was on the left towards the center where his hand now covered his own head. Linking the details of the headache to the details of the trauma provided an organizational structure on which Lee could lean. Perhaps there was meaning in his various forms of suffering. Thus, it contributed to the developing working alliance.

It was another somatic symptom which ultimately carried the central configuration of Lee's trauma in Vietnam. And it was not until much later in the treatment that it emerged. For some time the therapist knew that Lee had been active in 'Operation Phoenix' during the Vietnam War. This was a complex project, in which the CIA apparently took an active role and which involved among other things systematic assassination and grotesque markings made on the bodies of leaders thought to be friendly to the other side. Lee complained of severe joint pains often when he found himself ruminating about a peace-time 'mission' against a current day 'enemy'. Pain was sharp and deep in the joints, affected mostly the shoulders but also the knees and at times the wrist and fingers. There was no redness, warmth, or swelling or point tenderness; there was usually multiple joint involvement over the course of several hours although at a single point in time it would appear only one joint to be most markedly affected. It took the therapist quite some time to be able to verbalize his understanding to the patient, namely that Lee had the task of dismembering the enemy in a ceremonial manner following certain of these assassinations. Like Josh, Lee had incorporated the somatic experience of his victim(s) into a persistent symptom of his own. As agent of the horror, Lee could neither grieve nor work through his complex feelings about these deaths, unconsciously preserving them within his own tortured soma. By decoding the message, the doctor could bridge the agony of Lee's guilt, and also help Lee define the central painful meaning of his trauma experience: a succumbing to and identification with the horror which surrounded him.

Summary of Clinical Findings

The patients described here who developed these posttrauma somatic symptoms were both men and women; they were victims, perpetrators and rescure workers in traumatic situations involving death; the symptoms had persisted anywhere from 6 months to 16 years; no physiologic system seemed immune. There were musculo-skeletal, genitourinary, cardiopulmonary, gastrointestinal and connective tissue involved. The stressor events encapsulated in these symptoms deal with grotesque death, such as an enemy ritually dismembered. Even the tag on the 17-year-old's heel is an eerie sight within the context of a gymnasium turned into a temporary morgue. The patients appeared in real duress. The specific symptoms *repeated actual memories* with uncanny precision. The repetition had the characteristics of a traumatic nightmare. It was like a flashback or intrusive image of trauma taking somatic form and hence would best be distinguished from conversion reaction and given its own name: a somatic reenactment.

Somatic Reenactment versus Conversion Reaction

Characteristically, a somatic reenactment mimics in fine detail an actual traumatic experience whereas the contours of a given conversion reaction tend to symbolize but *not* reproduce an actual experience. For example Lee's unusually demarcated headache, exactly reproducing the outlines of the rifle butt impression against the Vietnam boy's head, contrasts with conversion paralysis of the right hand taking form in an overwhelmed mother just before she was about to strike her child with it. A conversion reaction requires *symbolic* connection to conflict or need; the somatic reenactment, like the traumatic nightmare, repeats the imagery of the trauma itself, with symbol formation developing secondarily. The clinician, in a conversion reaction, must identify a conflict which is convincingly expressed by the compromise of the physical symptom. The clinician, in a somatic reenactment, must establish the traumatic memory which continues unmetabolized by the psyche, and persists in returning via this intrusive form. 'La belle indifférence', which is sometimes present in conversion reactions, is typically absent in somatic reenactments: i.e. patients clearly complain and suffer from their physical symptoms sometimes to the point of anguish.

Finally, it is striking that in most cases the somatic symptom did not repeat what happened to the *survivor* but rather it repeated what happened to an intimate victim. Mrs. F. imagined that her friends had felt urinary urgency and therefore had excused themselves to the lavatory. It was not Lee's head or joints which had received injury in the war but rather it was his victim's in life an death struggles in which he was the survivor. Such a mechanism is analogous to Freud's description of a hysterical identification with the lost object [11].

The interactive process in which this discovery regarding the somatic reenactment was made between patient and doctor had several features in common. In each case, there was mutuality in arriving at this explanation, both the patient and the doctor seemed near the same conclusion at the same time. For the doctor this was often with a sense of revelation; for the patient the insight failed to have the intensity of a memory which has been removed from repression. But rather it was a memory that the patient knew was there all the time. It was more in the area of disavowal than unconscious denial. Hence, the discovery was experienced by the patient more as relief than revelation: now finally someone might understand. The resulting psychoeconomic shifts following interpretation varied with the different patients and different phases of treatment. In general, there was a freeing up of energy previously sequestered in the somatic symptom. But the readiness to reengage grief and mourning varied. For the priest and Mrs. F. at the fire, interpretation activated mourning as it did for Josh, but Lee's role as agent was more profound and the psychic pain associated with memory at times seemed even greater than the somatic pain of his reenactment.

Group Level Quantitative Findings

Like many trauma investigators in the 1980s, we did not design our studies with special attention directed to somatic features of PTSD. However, two preexisting somatic subscales were already part of the battery of self-report and clinician-based instruments we were using and offered us some general group level observations. The Psychiatriy Evaluation Form [12] is rated by clinical interviewers, on a 1–6 scale. One of the 19 dimensions is the degree to which the subject expresses emotional distress in somatic terms, not explainable by concurrent physical illness. Ratings of 1 and 2 are typical of nonpatient populations, 3 and 4 typical of outpatients and 5 and 6 more like inpatients.

The Symptom Checklist-90 [13], a self-report scale of clinical distress, has a standardized 12-item somatic subscale, with the items rated on a (0–4) scale for intensity. Symptoms on this scale include items such as headache, dizziness, chest pain, nausea, muscle soreness, and numbness or tingling. Scores on these scales have been reported by our group and others on civilian posttrauma samples, psychiatriy outpatients and on nonpatient control groups, and are available for comparison purposes.

In general somatic distress, in the several survivor populations we studied, correlated with the extent of the traumatic stressor (e.g. bereavement, threat to life, etc.). The cases presented here were all part of larger group level studies of trauma survivors. Survivors of war and civilian catastrophe who presented clinically, scored at the level of other psychiatric outpatients. But overlapping domains among subscales on each of these measures is considerable, and a separate effect for the somatic subscales could not be documented.

A small treatment sample of Vietnam veterans who presented initially whith somatic complaints, as expected scored notably higher on somatic subscales than nonclinical Vietnam veterans and slightly higher on these scales than the total treatment sample.

Those whose somatic distress was connected with somatic reenactment, as in the cases above, improved notably during treatment especially on the PEF somatic subscale; while those whose somatic symptoms were attributed to an *Agent Orange Syndrome*[1], got worse (numbers too small for significance). In the latter instance, understanding the meaning of the symptoms increased risk of future medical illness and possible genetic damage. This simply fueled rage rather than integrating split-off and disavowed affect.

Further group level studies on the rates and types of somatic symptoms present with PTSD are called for and special clinical attention should be addressed to somatic reenactments as a special form of somatic symptom amenable to a psychotherapeutic approach.

[1] *'Agent Orange'* is a toxic defoliant used in Vietnam to clear otherwise hidden supply routes. It contains dioxin, a highly potent toxin reported to cause chronic chloracne and birth defects.

References

1 Kardiner A: Traumatic neurosis of war; in Arieti S (ed): American Handbook of Psychiatry, 1959, pp 245–257.

2 Eitinger L: Pathology of the concentration camp syndrome. Arch Psychiatry 1961;5:79–87.

3 Titchener JT, Kapp F: Family and character change at Buffalo Creek. Am Psychiatry 1976;133:295–299.

4 Carden N, Schramel D: Observations of conversion reactions seen in troops involved in the Vietnam conflict. Am J Psychiatry 1966;123:21–30.

5 Kadushin C, Boulanger G, Smith JR: Long-term stress reactions: Some causes, consequences, and naturally occurring support systems (Appendix 1A: The stress scales); in Egendorf A, Kadushin C, Laufer RS, Rothbart G, Sloan L (eds): Legacies of Vietnam. Washington, US Government Printing Office, 1981, pp 651–664.

6 Solomon Z, Mikuliner M: Combat stress reactions, posttraumatic stress disorder and somatic complaints among Israeli soldiers. J Psychosom Res 1987;31:131–137.

7 Solomon Z, Mikulineer M, Kolter M: A two-year follow-up of somatic complaints among Israeli combat stress reaction casualties. J Psychosom Res 1987;31:463–469.

8 Shalev A, Beleich A, Ursano R: Post-traumatic stress disorder: Somatic comorbidity and effort tolerance. Presentation at Annu Meet Soc Traumatic Stress Studies, Dallas, 1988.

9 Centers for Disease Control: Health status of Vietnam veterans. II Physical health. JAMA 1988;259:2708–2714.

10 Lindy JD: An outline for the psychoanalytic psychotherapy of post traumatic stress disorder; in Figley CR (ed): Trauma and Its Wake, II: Traumatic Stress Theory, Research, and Intervention. New York Brunner/Mazel 1986.

11 Freud S: Mourning and Melancholia, standard ed; in Strachey J (ed): Freud's Completed Works. London, Hogarth, 1917, vol 18, pp 249–251.

12 Spitzer R, Endicott J, Mesnikoff A, Cohen M: The Psychiatric Evaluation Form. New York, Biometrics Research, 1968.

13 Derogatis L: R Version Manual J (SCL-90). Baltimore, Johns Hopkins University, 1977.

2nd Europ Conf on Traumatic Stress
Psychother Psychosom 1992;57:187–193

Tom Lundin
Ulf Otto

Department of Psychiatry
University Hospital of Linköping,
Sweden

Swedish UN Soldiers in Cyprus, UNFICYP: Their Psychological and Social Situation

Key Words
UN Service
Cyprus
Military psychiatry
Stress reactions
Posttraumatic stress disorder

Abstract
Two Swedish rifle batallions serving as UN soldiers in Cyprus (UNFICYP) have been investigated with respect to their demographic background and motives for application for UN service. The comparison of symptoms of stress in general, of posttraumatic stress disorder specifically, and some other variables of reaction with various studies of Swedish UN soldiers in different settings has given the following results. Very few interviewees experienced 'personal nervous breakdown' (0.5%). The soldiers reported in general very few psychological or psychosomatic complaints in the short time perspective. There seemed, however, to be two groups of persons at risk, namely those who were repatriated and those with a high consumption of alcohol.

Introduction

Since 1948 more than 60,000 Swedish men and women have been in military UN service in more than 15 countries under very different circumstances [1]. The stress situations for UN soldiers are different according to the political and military situations. The UNEF (United Nation Emergency Force) was partly a Swedich mission during the years 1957–1961. The UNEF area consisted of the Gaza Strip and the Sinai Peninsula. The Swedish battalion was around 1,000 men. The mean value for annual repatriations was 0.76%. Only 11 cases of psychiatric disorders resulted in repatriation. The total number of mental cases admitted to UNEF Hospital during these 5 years was 138, 59% of these were repatriated [2]. The combat strain of 1,086 Swedish soldiers serving the UN forces in Congo 1961–1962 has been studied [3] and compared with 1,242 Swedish UN soldiers, who were noncombat veterans. The combat veterans did not differ from the noncombat veter-

Tom Lundin, MD, PhD
University Hospital of Linköping
S–581 85 Linköping (Sweden)

0033–3190/92/
0574–0187$2.75/0

ans in total morbidity or psychiatric morbidity after their UN service. The combat veterans were however significantly more prone to accidents during the first few years after their service. There were no differences in number of alcohol offences after the UN service. There were only 35 soldiers in total, who developed 'combat exhaustion' (posttraumatic stress disorder, PTSD). The soldiers who broke down more often had parents with a psychiatric history, came more often from broken homes, and were of lower intellectual level, on average, than those who did not break down.

The psychological situation for the UN soldier is quite different from soldiers in other military situations [4, 5]. He has to carefully control his reactions when provoked. The UN soldier might be scared by his own aggressiveness, because of his limited possibilities to use his weapons. The total number of reported psychiatric cases, including repatriations in all 11 national contingents that participated in UNIFIL from April 1978 to August 1980 has been studied [6, 7]. It was found that the psychiatric morbidity of the total forces was low, 0.9% (n = 394). The frequency of repatriations due to mental problems was low (n = 98) during the whole period [8]. A number of 74 of the UNIFIL personnel were in addition treated as out-patients for various psychiatric disorders at the UNIFIL hospital [9].

The drinking habits of the soldiers of one of the Norwegian contingents have been studied. It was found that the average consumption of alcohol was 0.32 liter calculated as pure alcohol per week, equivalent to 1 liter of liquor [5]. This represented a considerable increase to the reported consumption before departure, and also over the mean consumption of 150 ml per week for the same age groups of Norwegian males.

In an earlier study stress reactions have been reported among Swedish health care personnel [10] as well as mental adjustment of one Swedish logistic battalion [11] in South Lebanon. In the first of these studies [10] three contingents (n = 421) were studied by help of questionnaires, self-rating-scales, personality inventory test and personal interviews. The personal interviews were structured and performed during the last month of service for each contingent. The UN soldiers were interviewed by 6 experienced psychiatrists. In the study of the logistic battalion a high proportion of stress symptoms was found as well as feelings of monotony.

Between the years 1964 and 1987 Sweden took part in the UN peace-keeping forces in Cyprus. The responsibility was one rifle battalion. The Swedish participation ceased 1987 mainly for economic reasons. During these 23 years more than 15,000 Swedish men and women were in UN service in UNFICYP, Cyprus. It was decided to study and follow up two battalions in order to get more knowledge on the specific stress factors for UN soldiers in this type of service. It was also important to improve the selection criteria, since the repatriation rate was too high.

Material and Methods

Two rifle battalions (n = 649) during the years 1984–1985 were studied by help of questionnaires before and after their UN service period, personal semistructured interviews performed by well educated and trained psychiatrists and self-rating scales. The personal interviews were structured and performed during the last month of the service period. The UN soldiers were interviewed by 6 experienced psychiatrists, who were all well acquainted with the Swedish military system. All the inteviews took place within the UN campus in Cyprus. For practical reasons it was not possible to personally interview 100% of the contingents because some people were on leave during the interview period. The questionnaires were based on those used in earlier studies on Swedish UN soldiers [10, 11]. *Significance testing* was done with help of Student's t test.

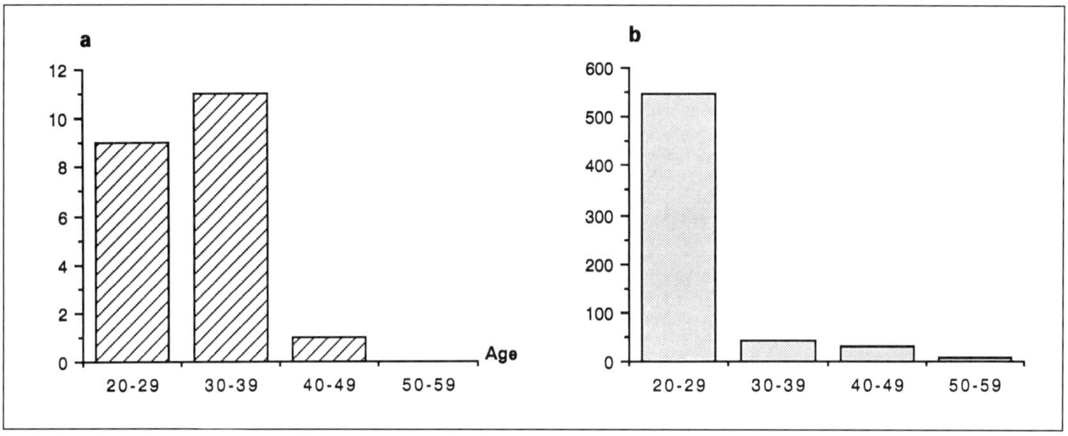

Fig. 1. UNFICYP, women (**a**) and men (**b**), distribution by age.

Results

The studied group included 21 women and 628 men, altogether 649 persons with a mean age of 27.2 years. The age distributions are shown in figure 1a, b. Only 13.3% of the soldiers came from the three big cities in Sweden, 25.4% from rural areas and the rest, 60.9% from smaller towns or communities. The *educational level* was relatively low (high = 6.0%; medium = 80.4%; low = 10.2%). Only around 16% were married or living together (table 1). Almost 60% had a civil employment before the UN service period. None of the 21 women were unemployed, but 12.1% of the men had no job to go back to after the service. Only 8.2% of the whole group were full-time military employees (table 2). The actual UN service period was the first one for 73.0% of the *interviewees* with a small difference between men and women (table 3). Only very few, less than 3%, reported more than one earlier service period. They were asked to indicate personal reasons for applying for UN service. The most important were change of milieu, economic advantages, to get abroad, good for one's own career, and searching for adventure (table 4).

Table 1. Civil status (%) before the present UN service

	UNIFIL (n = 241)		UNFICYP (n = 649)	
	male	female	male	female
Married or living together	24.4	20.8	16.8	15.8

It has been supposed that one of the most important background variables which might determine the ability to cope with the specific stress factors of the military situation is the training and preparation for the mission. Almost 90% of the whole group estimated their *education* as good or moderate on a three-degree scale (table 5). The subjectively experienced incidence of 'nervous breakdown' was extremely low, 0.5%. There seemed to be good possibilities for personal support by fellows and friends, 77.4% of the respondents.

Table 2. Civil employment, UNFICYP, before the present UN service (in %, n = 649)

	Male (n = 628)	Female (n = 21)	Total (n = 649)
Medical service or health care	4.1	19.0	4.6
Military employment	8.3	4.8	8.2
Unemployed	12.1	0	11.7
Civil employment	59.6	66.7	59.8
No answer	15.9	9.5	15.7

Table 3. Number and frequency of respondents, UNFICYP; with earlier UN service experiences (n = 649)

Numer of earlier UN sevices	Male		Female		Total	
	n	%	n	%	n	%
0	456	72.6	18	85.7	474	73.0
1	59	9.4	1	4.8	60	9.2
2	10	1.6	0	–	10	1.5
3	1	0.2	0	–	1	0.2
4	2	0.3	1	4.8	3	0.5
5	–	–	–	–	–	–
6	–	–	–	–	–	–

Table 4. Reasons (in %) of the sample for applying for UN service in UNIFIL and UNFICYP (the respondents have given more than one reason).

Item	UNIFIL (n = 360)	UNFI CYP (n = 624)
Difficulies in getting a job	5.8	8.7
Get away from problems and difficulties at home	0.6	1.1
Relation problems	0.6	0.3
Getting on badly with work	4.2	6.1
Feelings of disgust at Swedish internal politics	6.4	5.4
Change of milieu	66.9	42.3
Thinking over one's own situation	3.3	7.5
Economic advantages	8.3	22.4
To get abroad	83.9	95.3
Good for one's own career	13.6	49.2
Searching for an adventure	35.3	55.6
Idealism	8.1	12.5

Table 5. Subjective estimation of the training and education for the UN service (in %) for men and women (UNFICYP)

Education and training before UN service	Sex		Total (n = 649)
	male (n = 628)	female (n = 21)	
Good	28.0	31.6	28.8
Moderate	61.0	47.4	60.5
Bad	8.5	15.8	8.8
No answer	2.5	5.2	1.9

Table 6. Differences between UNIFIL and UNFICYP between some variables of reaction (in %)

Item	UNIFIL (n = 340)	UNFICYP (n = 649)	p
Subjective estimation of 'personal nervous breakdown'	5.6	0.5	< 0.001
Possibilities for personal support	82.9	77.4	NS
Too high use of alcohol (self-rated)	24.7	9.6	< 0.001
Considered leaving UN service	19.2	9.0	< 0.001
Feelings of monotony at work	51.3	63.6	< 0.001
Homesickness for age group 20–29	53.1	30.7	< 0.001

Table 7. Some symptoms and reactions related to stress (in %) of a self-rating scale (often/sometimes)

Item	UNIFIL (n = 340)	UNFICYP (n = 605)	p
Depression	9.4	8.6	NS
Sleep disturbances	7.1	6.6	NS
Nightmares	1.2	1.5	NS
Anxiousness/ restlessness	10.6	13.7	< 0.05
A need for isolation	24.1	16.2	< 0.001
Unpleasant feelings at work	7.1	7.6	NS
Muscular tension	1.5	1.2	NS

Less than 10% of the whole group estimated their consumption of alcohol to be too high.

Around 30% of the *interviewees* had intensive or moderate feelings of homesickness, but less than ten per cent considered from time to time leaving the service before the end of the period (table 6). A relatively high proportion of the group experienced their situation to be monotonous.

Stress Symptoms

Some stress symptoms and reactions, such as depression, sleep disturbances, nightmares, and muscular tension were low in incidence. Anxiousness and a need for isolation were the only symptoms that were reported by more then 10% of the studied group. There were no significant differences between men and women (table 7).

Discussion

The stress reactions among the soldiers of two specialized UN military units, the medical company and a logistic battalion, have been described [10, 11]. Since the present study has been carried out with the same method and the same instruments as the study on the psychological and psychosocial situation of three UNIFIL medical companies [10] it was possible to compare the present findings with the earlier ones. In an earlier study [10] we presented the special situation for a UN soldier including the stress effects of (1) staying in a military camp far away from home; (2) the combat strain, and (3) the limited possibilities to use one's own weapons. The psychiatric morbidity among UN soldiers is expected to be much lower than for the population in general according to the selection criteria, which in Sweden have been developed by the Swedish Army, UN office, during the last 3 decades. By using the very strict inclusion criteria, the aim has been to exclude unsuitable applicants.

The soldiers of the UNFICYP rifle battalion were markedly younger (mean age 27.2 years) than the members of the UNIFIL medical company (mean age 39.1 years). The low educational level as well as the lower proportion of people married or living together (table 1) compared with the UNIFIL group might be explained by the lower mean age. Concerning the job situation, the most striking difference between the UNIFIL and UNFICYP soldiers was the frequency of unemployment, which is probably also an effect of the age factor. Very few had any earlier experiences of UN service, since most of the rifle soldiers in the UNIFICYP group were around the age of 25. Age-related differences were reported among the reasons for applying for UN service.

The older soldiers of UNIFIL were more interested to have a change in milieu and less in economic advantages. The younger ones of UNFICYP seemed to be in search for adventure and thought the service period might be good to their career.

According to this study the specialized education and training of *The UN School of the Swedish Army* seemed to be efficient for the actual mission in Cyprus. The females were more critical, probably depending on the fact that they had no previous military experience. They were therefore less well prepared for the military milieu during their UN service.

There were also some distinct differences between the two units concerning some variables of reaction (table 6). The medical personnel scored significantly higher on most variables except feeling of montony at work. Earlier studies [10, 11] have shown that UN soldiers in general are monotony avoiders. The selection criteria for the UNIFIL personnel had to be quite different from those for UNFICYP according to their tasks. A great many persons of the medical company had the same or similar tasks as in their ordinary civilian employment. They might, however, at the same time, through personal and professional contacts with wounded local civilians, have come closer to the reality of war than the rifle soldiers in Cyprus. The only stress symptoms that scored significantly different for the two groups were anxiousness and a need for isolation (table 7). These differences might as well be an effect of age as an effect of different political and social circumstances for the mission and different tasks. The situation for the UNFICYP soldier was also much more free and open than it was in the relatively small UNIFIL camp with its psychologically more obtrusive atmosphere. This might also explain the higher scoring for homesickness in Lebanon compared with Cyprus. It was also easier for family members to travel to Cyprus with tourist-groups and to visit the soldiers at the camp.

Conclusions

The present study together with the earlier studies on Swedish UN soldiers [10, 11] show that the Swedish selection criteria for UN service, education, and training seem to be adequate at least for these three missions. The soldiers of the studied groups had no combat experiences. They developed few psychological or psychosomatic problems in the short time perspective. There were, however, in all three groups persons at risk (e.g. cases of repatriation and heavy drinkers), who might develop psychosocial problems or psychiatric disorders with a delayed onset.

References

1 Otto U (ed): Katastrof- och försvarspsykiatri. Lund, Studentlitteratur, 1986.
2 Kluge T, Lønnum A, Udjus L: Diseases in the UNEF troops 1956–1961/62. Rev Int Services Santé 1963;(suppl 5):26–46.
3 Kettner B: Combat strain and subsequent mental health. A follow-up study of Swedish soldies serving in the United Nations forces 1961–62. Acta Psychiatr Scand 1972 (suppl 230).
4 Weisaeth L: Stressmedicinske erfaringer fra UNIFIL. Sanitetsnytt, 1979;October:83–97.
5 Weisaeth L: Psykiatri og stress hos FN-soldater i Syd-Libanon. (stencil). Oslo, Psyckiatrisk Institutt. 1979.
6 Weisaeth L, Sund A: Psychiatric problems in UNIFIL and the UN soldier's stress syndrome. Rev Int Service Santé, 1982;55:109–116.
7 Lønnum A, Kluge T, Malm OJ: Health and disease in UNIFIL. Rev Int Service Santé 1982;55:52–68.
8 Hesla PE, Malm OJ: Repatriations of UNIFIL personnel. Rev Int Services Santé, 1982;55:75–78.
9 Gude H, Johnsen PG: UNIFIL hospital. Rev Int Services Santé 1982; 55:79–92.
10 Lundin T, Otto U: Stress reactions among Swedish health care personnel in UNIFIL, South Lebanon 1982–1984. Stress Med 1989;5: 237–246.
11 Carlström A, Lundin T, Otto U: Mental adjustment of Swedish UN soldiers in South Lebanon in 1988. Stress Med 1990;6:305–310.

2nd Europ Conf on Traumatic Stress
Psychother Psychosom 1992;57:194–199

Piet R. Wiepkema
Willem G.P. Schouten

Department of Animal Husbandry, Section Ethology, Agricultural University at Wageningen, The Netherlands

Stereotypies in Sows during Chronic Stress

Key Words
Chronic stress
Stereotypies
Coping styles

Abstract
In pig husbandry sows are fixed in such a way that they undergo a chronic loss of control over their environment. In these conditions sows develop stereotypies that are associated with a specific activation of brain endorphins. Stereotyping itself reduces some neuroendocrine stress symptoms. During stress at least two coping styles can be distinguished in many mammals and birds. These types are found again in the stressed sows which either maintain a high or a low level of stereotypies. The low stereotyping sows show the strongest signs of uneasiness.

Introduction

In present-day pig husbandry in Western Europe most pregnant sows are tied up for months (pregnancy period) by means of a neck or a breast tether (fig. 1). This tethering, based on dubious economic arguments, fixes each individual to one place and makes it part of rows of other sows kept in the same stall. In this position a sow cannot freely explore its surroundings, it cannot defecate at a location different from where it has to lie down, it cannot make or break specific social contacts, and finally it can only wait for its food and water. Without doubt such animals experience a substantial loss of control over relevant environmental aspects during about 3–4 successive months. For sows that are as keen and as social as, for instance, many domestic dogs, this type of housing represents a dramatic and long-lasting interference with their natural lifestyle. However, most of these sows survive. How do sows cope with this chronic stress condition? In this contribution we will review some relevant behavioral and physiological aspects of their coping, since the findings involved may have general significance for an understanding of comparable processes that take place in vertebrates, including men, during a chronic loss of control (stress).

P.R. Wiepkema
Dept. of Animal Husbandry, Section Ethology
Agricultural University at Wageningen
Postbox 338
NL-6700 AH Wageningen (The Netherlands)

0033–3190/92/
0574–0194$2.75/0

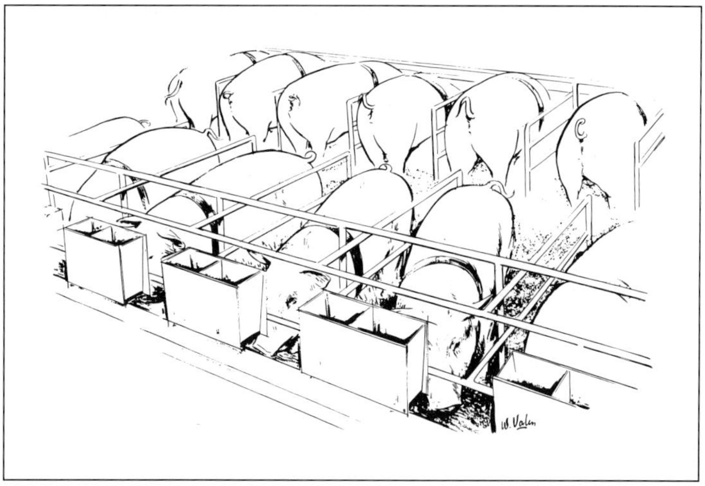

Fig. 1. Two rows of breast-tethered sows. The tether has been fixed with a chain to the floor. One of the two food boxes in front of each sow is opened once or twice a day. Only then the sow can eat a restricted amount of food.

Tethered Sows

Just over a week after a successful insemination, sows are stalled in rows and tethered. About 3 months later the pregnant sow is moved to a farrowing crate, where she is tethered or fixed again. In this crate the litter is born and the piglets remain for about 4 weeks with the mother. Thereafter the dry sow is inseminated as soon as possible and the whole cycle starts again. Most sows produce only 2 or 3 litters, since for various reasons (for instance, not showing estrous signs again), many sows have to be removed prematurely. The animals are fed a commercial diet and watered once or twice a day: the diet is presented in a trough, while the water is available via a nipple. Most of the data to be presented here stem from such practice conditions.

To fasten an inseminated sow she is lured with some food in her future stand and, while eating, she is fixed with, for instance, a neck tether. After finishing her small meal and discovering her fixed position, the sow tries to break out by pulling and biting at the chain (of the neck tether) and/or by pushing fiercely against the wall and bars that are in front of her. This initial breakout behavior is often, but not always, very intensive in the first hours of being tethered. Sometimes a sow may even free herself: such sows are difficult to fasten again. After this first resistance the breakout behavior undergoes some changes: (1) it becomes less intensive; (2) gradually it is repeated over and again, and (3) it becomes ritualized, that is, the original behavior becomes simpler, more stereotyped and typical for the individual [1, 2].

These changes take place in the course of some weeks (but this differs from individual to individual); the resulting behavior patterns are called stereotypies. These stereotypies are characterized by the following: (1) they are repeated over and again; (2) they have a relatively constant form; (3) they seem to serve no obvious goal, and (4) they are idiosyncratic. A representative example of such a stereotypy of tethered sows is the following sequence of behavioral elements: chewing the chain, chewing while the mouth is empty, licking the trough, chewing the chain again, etc. The duration of each cycle, consisting of 3 different elements, is very constant. It makes sense to dis-

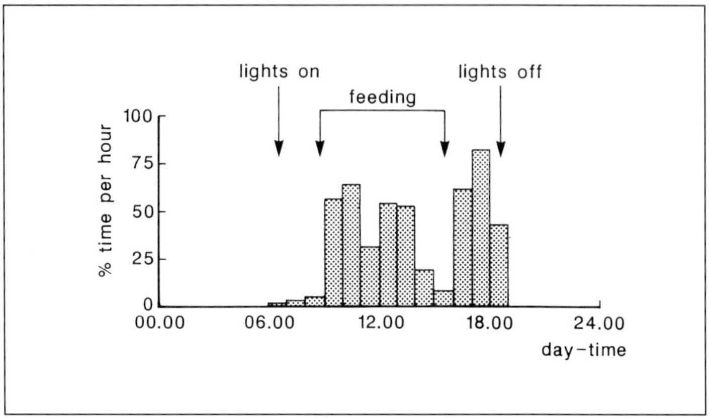

Fig. 2. Ordinate: time spent in performing stereotypies during a 24-hour period. During the night hours (from 18.30 until 07.00 h) the sows rest and do not perform stereotypies.

tinguish these stereotypies from normal stereotyped routine behavior used to obtain food, to clean oneself, etc. that serves obvious goals.

The stereotypies of tethered sows dominate in the periods after feeding time (fig. 2) and are different from the stereotyped behavior the animals show just before feeding [3]. These latter routines can best be conceived as operants the animal sees as necessary and successful actions to obtain food: in fact it is superstitious behavior. The characteristics of the presented stereotypies are: (1) they mainly occur just after feeding and (2) the amount of stereotypy performance differs enormously between sows; some spend up to 10 h per day in stereotyping, others at the most 1 h [1].

Stereotypies in Other Vertebrates

Behavior patterns that meet the above-mentioned criteria for stereotypies are not uncommon in mammals and birds that for longer periods of time are kept inadequately. The following examples may illustrate this. Milk-fed veal calves develop a stereotyped rolling up and unrolling of the tongue that is called tongue-playing [4]; it results from the absence of roughage (grass, hay, straw) the calves need to develop rumination. Separately stalled horses may perform hours of swaying with the head (weaving); its causation is not quite clear [5]. The same holds for zoo-bound polar bears that with awful precision step when moving up and down in their enclosure. Cage-kept mink spend much time in turning with their head and/or body around parts of their cage (for instance, the drink nipple) in a very rapid fashion and each in its own mode [6]. Canaries may perform a repeated jumping to and fro, when their cages are too small [7].

All these housing systems have one thing in common: the enclosures the animals live in prevent them from controlling relevant aspects of their environment by means of performing species-specific behavior. This chronic loss of control is typical of chronic stress [8] and can best be described as a state of uncertainty. This uncertainty has been associated with those life events that no longer can be controlled and is all the severer the more relevant these events are. Under such conditions mammals and birds develop at least two types of disturbed behavior: (1) stereotypies and (2) injurious behavior by which they damage themselves or animals of the same species [9]. In the following we will focus on the stereotypies only.

Stereotypies: Their Significance

The endless repetitions and the intensity with which the tethered sows perform their postfeeding stereotypies suggest some form of addiction. Therefore we investigated whether or not a specific endorphin antagonist could influence the occurrence of these stereotypies in a specific way. To do so we injected the tethered sows with saline or a saline-naloxone solution (1 mg naloxone per kg pig, i.m.) just after feeding [10]. We also injected free sows that could explore individually an unfamiliar pen with interesting objects (tree branch, some ground etc.). It turned out that naloxone strongly reduced the occurrence of stereotypies and only weakly (but significantly) the occurrence of exploratory behavior [8]. Cronin [1] reported that naloxone seems to have less effect on older (used for a long time) stereotypies. This idea was substantiated by the work of Kennes et al. [11] on stereotypies in voles. This reduced effect of naloxone may indicate a process of emancipation of the stereotypy itself in becoming loosened from its original underlying opioid mechanisms. In this context the findings of Panksepp et al. [12] may be relevant: these authors suggest a significant role for opioids in the early phase of the development of normal social behavior.

Although the β-endorphin plasma level may become high on the day sows are tethered (fig. 3), this level returns to normal or even subnormal on the following days and weeks, when the stereotypies are formed. It is most interesting that such subnormal plasma levels have been reported also in autistic children [13]. These low plasma levels and the existing responsiveness to naloxone indicate that brain endorphins are critical in the development of stereotypies. Present research is directed at this point. A plausible second role of these endorphins is that they directly or indirectly, in association with performing specific behavior, facilitate a calming down of the severely stressed sows. The indirect contribution is likely, because various reports [14–16] reveal a calming down effect of performing some behavior when being stressed or punished. This phenomenon is also reflected in our finding [unpubl. results] that tethered sows performing many stereotypies have a lower heart rate than those that perform few stereotypies.

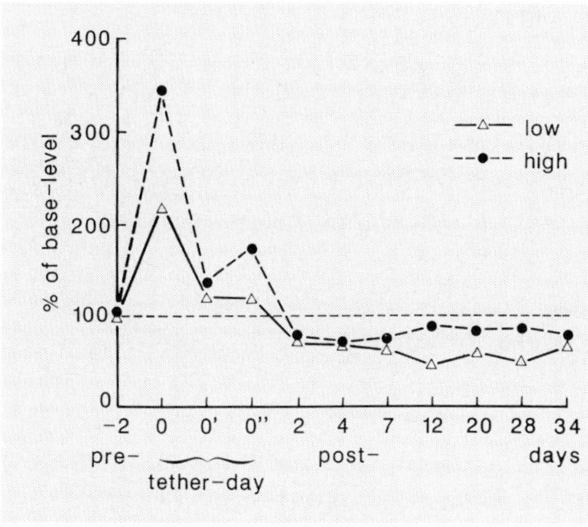

Fig. 3. Percentage of plasma base level β-endorphin 2 days before tethering, on the tether day (0 = just after tethering; 0′ = 20 min later, 0″ = 60 min later) and on a number of days after tethering). Base level of β-endorphin = 3 pmol/l. The data of two sows (with high or low endorphin levels at tethering) are shown.

The relationship between stereotypies and endorphins made us conjecture that performing stereotypies would increase analgesia. To test this we measured tail flick latency of tethered sows when a heated resistor (65 °C) was placed on their rump [17]. To our surprise it came out that pain sensitivity was highest (and possibly nearest to normal) in those animals that performed most stereotypies. To explain this unexpected association we think that performing many stereotypies not only calms down but also restores normal capabilities and responsiveness for those aspects that are not directly connected with tethering as such. To understand this more completely we have to say some words about individual differences in coping styles.

Styles of Coping

A most important point in present-day studies is that individuals of the same species, gender and age appear to cope in either a predominantly sympathetic or a parasympathetic way [18]. An interesting illustration of the existence of two coping styles has been found for veal calves that were fed with milk only [19]. As stated before such calves develop tongue-playing, a stereotypy. However, not all calves do so with the same intensity. We found that those calves that developed much tongue-playing did not show stomach wall (pyloric) ulcers when slaughtered at the age of 20 weeks. Calves that did not develop tongue-playing all had such ulcers at the same slaughter age. Our tethered sows also showed different coping styles in that all sows could be categorized into two separate groups: sows that spent much time on stereotypies and sows that spent little time behaving in the same way. These two groups were significantly different with respect to their analgesia [17] and their average heart rate [heart rate being highest in the low-stereotyping sows; unpubl. results]. Most interesting is the following recent finding [20]. Since we thought that the tethered sows which show many stereotypies represent an extrovert type of individuals in contrast to those that perform few stereotypies, we expected that the first category of sows would show the highest overt resistance at the first tethering day. This was not what we found. The picture is unambiguous and as follows: intensive initial resistance is associated with a low stereotyping level later on. This surprising negative and highly significant correlation between level of initial resistance and level of later stereotypy performance leads to the conclusion that those animals (the sympathetic ones?) that try to break out fiercely and desperately, evaluate their position as helpless and develop some form of passive resignation. On the other hand those animals that only weakly try to break out are able to develop a behavioral strategy (stereotypies) that significantly reduces relevant chronic stress symptoms (heart rate, analgesia). From this point of view the low-stereotyping sows are in a worse condition than the high-stereotyping ones. However, both types of reaction are clearcut examples of disturbed animal welfare.

Conclusion

During chronic stress, that is, during a chronic loss of control over relevant environmental events, sows react by performing stereotypies. The form and level of these stereotypies are typical of the individual. These stereotypies may have a significant calming down effect, but not all animals are able to develop such behavior. These findings in sows may present a more general picture of the way mammals (including men) and birds cope with chronic stressors. In sows we know that such chronic stress is associated with reduced reproductive capacity and a reduced immune response [21].

References

1 Cronin GM: The development and significance of abnormal stereotyped behavior in tethered sows; PhD thesis, Agricultural University Wageningen, 1985.

2 Stolba A, Baker N, Wood-Gush DGM: The characterization of stereotyped behavior in stalled sows by information redundancy. Behaviour 1983;87:157–182.

3 Rushen J: Stereotyped behaviour, adjunctive drinking and the feeding periods of tethered sows. Anim Behav 1989;32:1059–1067.

4 Sambraus HH: Mouthbased anomalous syndromes; in Fraser AF (ed): World Animal Science 5. Ethology of Farm Animals. Amsterdam, Elsevier, 1985, pp 391–422.

5 Sambraus HH: Stereotypies; in Fraser AF (ed): World Animal Science 5. Ethology of Farm Animals. Amsterdam, Elsevier, 1985, pp 431–441.

6 De Jonge G, Carlstead K, Wiepkema PR: Das Wohlbefinden von Farmnerzen. Göttingen, Echo-Verlag, 1987, pp 1–54.

7 Keiper R: Causal factors of stereotypies in caged birds. Anim Behav 1969;17:114–119.

8 Wiepkema PR: Stress: Ethological implications; in Puglisi-Allegra S, Oliverio A (eds): Psychobiology of Stress. Dordrecht, Kluwer, 1990, pp 1–13.

9 Wiepkema PR, Broom DM, Duncan IJH, van Putten G: Abnormal behaviour in farm animals, CEC-Report Brussel, 1983, 1–16.

10 Cronin GM, Wiepkema PR, van Ree JM: Endorphins implicated in stereotypies of tethered sows. Experientia 1986;42:198–199.

11 Kennes D, Ödberg FO, Bouquet Y, de Rycke PH: Changes in naloxone and haloperidol effects during the development of captivity-induced jumping stereotypy in bank voles. Eur J Pharmacol 1988;153:19–24.

12 Panksepp J, Herman BH, Vilberg T, Bishop P, De Eskinazi FG: Endogenous opioids and social behaviour. Neurosci Biobehav Rev 1980;4: 473–487.

13 Weizman R, Weizman A, Tyano S, Szekely G, Weissman BA, Saryne Y: Humoral-endorphin blood levels in autistic, schizophrenic and healthy subjects. Psychopharmacology 1984;82:368–370.

14 Dantzer R, Mormède P: De-arousal properties of stereotyped behaviour: Evidence from pituitary-adrenal correlates in pigs. Appl Anim Ethol 1983;10:233-244.

15 Levine S, Weinberg J, Brett LP: Inhibition of pituitary-adrenal activity as a consequence of consummatory behaviour. Psychoneuroendocrinology 1979;4:275–286.

16 Levine S, Coe C, Wiener SG: Psychoneuroendocrinology of stress: A psychobiological perspective; in Brush FR, Levine S (eds): Psychoneuroendocrinology. San Diego, Academic Press, 1989, pp 341–377.

17 Rushen J, de Passillé AM, Schouten WGP: Stereotypic behavior, endogenous opioids, and postfeeding hypoalgesia in pigs. Physiol Behav 1990;48:91–96.

18 Bohus B, Benus RF, Fokkema DS, Koolhaas JM, Nyakas C, van Oortmerssen GA, Prins AJA, de Ruiter AJH, Scheurink AJW, Steffens AB: Neuro-endocrine states and behavioral and physiological stress responses. Progr Brain Res 1987;72: 57–70.

19 Wiepkema PR, van Hellemond KK, Roessingh P, Romberg H: Behaviour and abnormal damage in individual veal calves. Appl Anim Sci 1987;18:257–268.

20 Schouten WGP, Wiepkema PR: Coping styles in tethered sows, Behav Processes, 1991;25:125–132.

21 Barnett JL, Hemsworth PH: The impact of handling and environmental factors on the stress response and its consequences in swine. Lab Anim Sci 1986;August:366–369.

2nd Europ Conf on Traumatic Stress
Psychother Psychosom 1992;57:200–205

William Yule

University of London Institute of Psychiatry, London, UK

Post-Traumatic Stress Disorder in Child Survivors of Shipping Disasters: The Sinking of the 'Jupiter'

Key Words
Post-traumatic stress disorder
Children
Disaster

Abstract
334 of over 400 children who survived the sinking of the cruise ship, Jupiter, in Athens harbour in October 1988 completed a battery of questionnaires 5–9 months later. Compared with age- and sex-matched controls, they show significantly higher scores on depression and anxiety. They also report more fears, particularly of stimuli related to the trauma. Overall, their scores on the Impact of Events Scale are as high as those reported by adults in other disasters. Follow-up studies a year after the accident reveal that nearly half the children meet the DSM-III-R criteria for PTSD. The usefulness of this screening battery is discussed. Some evidence for the effects of early intervention in schools is presented.

Introduction

Children have been direct victims and survivors in many recent mass transport disasters. They are also the indirect victims in those where their relatives have been killed. There are few systematic studies of the effects of major trauma on children, and most of the published ones suffer major methodological weaknesses [1]. Garmezy and Rutter [2] concluded that severe, acute stressors such as occur in major disasters result in socially handicapping emotional disorders in some children, in the majority of cases the disturbances are short-lived. Because there were no reports of children showing amnesia for the traumatic event, nor showing 'psychic numbing' or intrusive flashbacks of the event, Garmezy and Rutter argued that there was no need for a specific diagnostic category for stress reactions in children parallel to the diagnostic category of post-traumatic stress disorder (PTSD) in adults. Thus conclusion is based on a lack of evidence [3]. The sort of broad-based behavioural rating screening instruments used in many early studies are simply not sen-

Professor William Yule
Institute of Psychiatry
de Crespigny Park
London SE5 8AF (UK)

0033–3190/92/
0574–0200$2.75/0

sitive to the subjective, intrusive thoughts and anxieties that many child victims experience. Teachers report less psychopathology among child survivors than do parents, and both report far less than the children themselves [3–6]. In studies carried out by the author and colleagues [3, 7], children reported very high levels of distressing, recurrent, intrusive thoughts on the Horowitz et al. [8] Impact of Events Scale. Pynoos et al. [9], in their study of the effects of a fatal shooting attack on children in a school playground in Los Angeles, also found that traumatized children can report their experiences through completing questionnaires. Children over 10 years of age have usually a very good understanding that their lives were threatened during a major disaster. Young teenagers often report a sense of foreshortened future. Teenagers who survived the Herald of Free Enterprise capsize often found it very hard to share their feelings with their parents. When child survivors of a mass transport disaster are scattered over many schools, there is, perhaps, more excuse for teachers being ill-prepared to deal with problems that manifest in the classroom. When children have returned from a traumatic school outing, there can be no such excuse. Children may well have enormous problems concentrating in class and in doing their homework. If they are not sleeping properly, all this gets exacerbated. Children are sensitized to a wide variety of stimuli, mention of which may trigger an emotional reaction, as in the child who had to read about the evacuation from Dunkirk. Teachers need to make arrangements for child survivors to leave the classroom when such events occur. Teachers need to be aware, too, of the reactions of other pupils towards the survivors.

This paper reports a large scale study of school-children who survived the sinking of a ship when they were on an educational cruise.

Method

Subjects. On October 21, 1988, the cruise ship Jupiter sailed from Athens with a party of nearly 400 British school-children and 90 teachers and parents aboard. They were setting out on a week's educational cruise of the eastern Mediterranean but were sunk by a tanker shortly after leaving harbour. One pupil, 1 teacher and 2 seamen were killed. Others were slightly hurt. Many children had to jump into the sea. Many were separated from their school parties for many hours. 5–9 months after the accident, solicitors acting for the children in pursuance of claims for personal injury asked all of them to complete a battery of questionnaires prepared by the author. A subsidiary study [13] has established that scores on this battery are good predictors of later help seeking among adolescent survivors. Although one must be concerned in case children pursuing litigation may exaggerate their distress, later detailed clinical examinations failed to reveal any such distortion. This is in accord with the observations in the Buffalo Creek disaster [15] where non-litigants were found to be *more* distressed than those suing for compensation. In all, forms were returned by 334 children – 76 boys and 258 girls. They ranged in age from 11 to 18 years, with most (64%) being aged 14 and 15 years, and therefore in their 2-year course of studies leading to the General Certificate of Secondary Education.

Measures. A modified form of the Fear Survey Schedule for Children [10] was used. This consisted of 98 items rated on a three-point scale. The Revised Children's Manifest Anxiety Scale [11] was selected as a measure of anxiety. The Birleson Depression Inventory [12] is an 18-item scale developed in Britain. Children rate symptoms on a three-point scale. Horowitz's Revised Impact of Events Scale [8] is a 15-item scale which measures the two most characteristic aspects of post-traumatic psychopathology, the strength of unpleasant, intrusive thoughts and the energy spent trying to block them out of consciousness.

Control Data. In a subsidiary study, 71 14-year-old girls from a school unaffected by the disaster also completed the battery, with the exception of the Impact of Events Scale, as they had experienced no traumatic event to rate. Normative data on 250 children aged 11–16 years were collected on the other measures in a parallel study [Yule et al., in preparation].

Table 1. Comparison of survivors and controls on measures of psychopathology

	Controls 124 boys/126 girls		Survivors 78 boys/256 girls		t	p
	mean	SD	mean	SD		
Depression						
Boys	7.76	4.14	9.41	5.27	2.33	<0.05
Girls	9.30	4.71	12.81	6.69	5.94	<0.01
Anxiety						
Boys	10.60	5.99	11.43	6.99	0.86	NS
Girls	12.40	6.14	15.11	7.31	3.81	<0.01
Unrelated fears						
Boys	14.06	6.80	15.49	8.42	1.20	NS
Girls	21.02	9.26	19.52	10.09	1.44	NS
Related fears						
Boys	4.11	2.84	8.16	5.31	5.84	<0.01
Girls	6.89	4.10	11.88	5.19	10.16	<0.01
Total fears (80 items)						
Boys	40.65	18.47	49.31	23.76	2.61	<0.01
Girls	57.54	22.71	63.67	25.91	2.36	<0.05
Impact of events						
Intrusion						
Boys	–		15.03	11.45		
Girls	–		18.21	9.77		
Avoidance						
Boys	–		14.32	11.09		
Girls	–		18.24	10.25		
Total						
Boys	–		29.34	20.95		
Girls	–		36.44	17.61		

Results

As can be seen in table 1, the traumatized children showed significantly higher scores on the measures of depression and girls, but not boys, showed significantly higher scores on anxiety. The total scores on the conventional 80-item part of the fear survey schedule significantly differentiated controls and affected children. Closer analysis revealed that the survivors showed significantly ($p < 0.01$) increased rates of fears related to stimuli present during the disaster, but not to unrelated stimuli. This is interpreted as supporting a conditioning model for the aetiology of these fears. On the Impact of Events Scale, the survivors score as high as adult survivors of other recent disasters. It is clear that intrusive thoughts and feelings are important and widespread reactions to major traumas among school children. On intrusive thoughts, avoidance, depression and anxiety, girls scored sig-

Table 2. Effects of early intervention in two girls schools

	Experimental school (n = 24)		Control school (n = 15)		t	p
	mean	SD	mean	SD		
Impact of events						
Intrusion	18.13	8.00	25.87	7.44	3.07	<0.01
Avoidance	17.58	8.28	23.13	10.06	1.79	(0.05)
Total	35.71	12.61	49.00	13.79	3.03	<0.01
Depression	14.17	6.00	16.00	8.19	0.75	NS
Anxiety	15.96	7.47	16.60	7.18	0.27	NS
Fears						
Related	10.88	5.05	13.87	4.73	1.87	(0.05)
Unrelated	19.32	8.71	25.00	7.23	2.20	<0.01
Total	62.50	23.29	74.00	19.35	1.67	(0.05)

p values in parentheses represent one-tailed values.

nificantly higher than boys. This is in keeping with findings in the literature on adults PTSD. In the present sample, there were no consistent age differences in reactions. There were significant differences in PTSD symptomatology across the different schools. Anecdotally, it was learned that different schools reacted to the disaster and its aftermath in different ways. Some quickly organized help from mental health professionals and were very supportive within the school. Others tried to ignore the whole episode and did not arrange any formal help. Eventually, it is hoped to get detailed accounts of what schools did do, but at the present time it is only possible to contrast the ratings at 5–9 months post-disaster in 2 girls schools with very different approaches. One school welcomed the offer of outside help; the other spurned it and the pupils got little systematic help until nearly a year after the disaster. In the school that accepted our help [13], we held a debriefing meeting for all the survivors 10 days after the disaster. Thereafter, we ran two small, open groups. We adopted a problem-solving approach, based on cognitive behavioural methods to target anxiety, avoidance and intrusive thoughts. In the contrasting school, no outside support was accepted until a year after the disaster. The data reported here were collected 5–9 months after it. As can be seen in table 2, on the self-report measures, pupils in the school that organized early intervention show significantly lower scores on the Impact of Events Scale, with the effect being stronger on the intrusion than on the avoidance items. Scores on the measures of Anxiety and Depression are slightly, but not significantly, lower. On the Fear Survey Schedule, girls in the actively treated school report significantly ($p < 0.05$, one-tailed) fewer fears overall, with the effect being stronger for unrelated than related fears.

Discussion

These results indicate that it is feasible to study the effects of disasters on adolescents using simple self-report scales. Such data can illuminate a number of issues relating to the effects of acute and traumatic stress on adolescents. In a detailed study of pupils in one school [7], it was found that exposure to the disaster was related to the levels of depression and anxiety, whereas fears were specifically increased only in those exposed. Yule and Udwin [13] showed that the battery of questionnaires given 10 days after the accident predicted psychopathology at 5 months, confirming Nader and Pynoos' [14] finding that PTSD in children is very stable at least across the 1st year. Over half the children were individually assessed 1 year after the accident and most of the high-risk group satisfied DSM-III-R criteria for PTSD. This means that approximately 50% of the child survivors had PTSD.

Treatment Needs

Our experience of working intensively with some of the Jupiter survivors has given us some insight into their treatment needs. In the immediate aftermath, children usually need to be reunited with their parents and family. Even teenagers may go back to sleeping in their parents' bed. Tolerance and understanding are called for. Survivors need to talk over what happened so as to get the sequence of events clear in their minds as well as to master the feelings that recall engenders.

Repetitive retelling is not enough alone. Professionals can help by creating a relatively safe environment in which such recounting can take place. Experiencing that the world does not come to an end when feelings are shared between parent and child can be very facilitating. Learning that other survivors share similar, irrational guilt about surviving can help to get things in perspective. Learning how to deal with anxiety attacks, how to identify trigger stimuli, how to take each day as it comes – all are important therapeutic tasks.

Implications for Treatment

The first need is to help children make sense of what happened to them and to gain mastery over their feelings. To this end, children should be treated in small groups. They should be asked to write detailed accounts of their experience and to be helped to cope with the emotions that brings up. In addition, they should be given specific treatment for fears, phobias and any other avoidant behaviours. They should get practical help with sleep disorders. Given that intrusive thoughts seemed worse at night just before dropping off to sleep, I advised many children to use portable tape recorders to play music to distract them and blot out the thoughts. With better sleep, they were better able to face the thoughts in the safety of daylight.

Conclusions

Events of recent years have forced on us an awareness of the emotional effects of disasters on children. It is clear that children as young as 8 years can suffer PTSD that is almost identical in form to that presented by adults. The effects can go on for 1–2 years, and cannot be considered transitory. Parents and teachers often underestimate the anxiety reactions that children report. Normal screening instruments will not pick up all the psychopathology.

There are developmental changes in children's reactions, but as so few young children have been studied, we cannot yet be clear of the nature of these changes. Children's reactions are intimately bound up with effects on the family, but some distress is directly caused by the trauma. Teachers, especially, need guidance on how to deal with the aftermath in schools. There is a great need for good treatment studies. Because disasters occur unexpectedly, we need to plan in advance how to conduct and evaluate all forms of intervention.

The present study has shown that adolescents can be screened using a battery measuring significant aspects of PTSD, depression and anxiety. Such a battery is potentially very useful in identifying children at high risk of developing PTSD following a mass disaster. Preliminary findings suggest that early intervention involving psychological debriefing, ongoing support for the teachers, group and individual treatment of the children is helpful in reducing reported levels of psychopathology.

Acknowledgements

I would like to thank the children, parents, teachers and solicitors for agreeing to let me use these data to increase our understanding of the effects of disasters on children. Earlier versions of this paper were presented to the 98th Annual Convention of the American Psychological Association, Boston, August 1990 and to the Second European Conference on Traumatic Stress, Noordwijkerhout, The Netherlands, September 1990. I am grateful to the Wellcome Foundation, the Tregaskis Bequest and the Herald Memorial Fund for financial support for the preparation of this paper.

References

1 Garmezy N: Children under severe stress: Critique and comments. J Am Acad Child Psychiatry 1986;25: 384–392.
2 Garmezy N, Rutter M: Acute reactions to stress; in Rutter M, Hersov L (eds): Child and Adolescent Psychiatry: Modern Approaches, ed 2, Oxford, Blackwell, 1985, pp 152–176.
3 Yule W, Williams R: Post traumatic stress reactions in children. J Trauma Stress 1990;3:279–295.
4 McFarlane AC, Policansky S, Irwin CP: A longitudinal study of the psychological morbidity in children due to a natural disaster. Psychol Med 1987;17:727–738.
5 Earls F, Smith E, Reich W, Jung KG: Investigating psychopathological consequences of a disaster in children: A pilot study incorporating a structured diagnostic approach. J Am Acad Child Psychiatry 1988;27:90–95.
6 Wolfe VV, Wolfe DA, Gentile C, LaRose L: Children's impact of traumatic events scale 1987; unpublished manuscript, University of Western Ontario, London, 1987.
7 Yule W, Udwin O, Murdoch K: The 'Jupiter' sinking: Effects on children's fears, depression and anxiety. J Child Psychol Psychiatry 1990;31: 1051–1061.
8 Horowitz MJ, Wilner N, Alvarez W: Impact of events scale: A measure of subjective stress. Psychosom Med 1979;41:209–218.
9 Pynoos RS, Frederick C, Nader K, Arroyo W, Steinberg A, Eth S, Nunez F, Fairbanks L: Life threat and post-traumatic stress in school-age children. Arch Gen Psychiatry 1987;44:1057–1063.
10 Ollendick TH, Yule W, Ollier K: Fears in British children and their relationship to manifest anxiety and depression. J Child Psychol Psychiatry 1991;32:321–331.
11 Reynolds CR, Richmond BO: What I think and feel: A revised measure of children's manifest anxiety. J Abnorm Child Psychol 1978;6:271–280.
12 Birleson P: The validity of depressive disorder in childhood and the development of a self-rating scale. J Child Psychol Psychiatry 1981;22: 73–88.
13 Yule W, Udwin O: Screening child survivors for post traumatic stress disorders: Experiences from the 'Jupiter' sinking. Br J Clin Psychol 1991;30:131–138.
14 Nader K, Pynoos RS, Fairbanks L, Frederick C: Childhood PTSD reactions one year after a sniper attack. Am J Psychiat 1990;146:1526–1530.
15 Gleser G, Green BL, Winget C: Prolonged psychosocial effects of disaster: A study of Buffalo Creek. New York, Plenum, 1981.

23rd Congress of the International Society of Psychoneuroendocrinology

Madison, Wisc., USA, August 16–20, 1992

Secretariat:

Ned H. Kalin, MD
Department of Psychiatry
University of Wisconsin Medical School
B6/210 Clinical Science Center
600 Highland Avenue
Madison, WI 53792 (USA)

1st Baltic Sea Conference on Psychosomatics and Psychotherapy

Kiel, FRG, September 16–19, 1992

Secretariat:

Klinik für Psychotherapie und Psychosomatik
Christian-Albrechts-Universität
Niemannsweg 147
D-W-2300 Kiel (FRG)

Author Index

(B) = Book Review

Subject Index

Vol. 57, 1992

Psychotherapy and Psychosomatics

Founded 1953 as 'Acta Psychotherapeutica et Psychosomatica'
by E.A.D.E. Carp and B. Stokvis, continued by
Th. Spoerri (1964–1974) and P.E. Sifneos (1974–1991)

KARGER

S. Karger
Medical and Scientific Publishers
Basel · Freiburg · Paris · London
New York · New Delhi · Bangkok
Singapore · Tokyo · Sydney

Drug Dosage
The authors and the publisher have exerted every effort to ensure that drug selection and dosage set forth in this text are in accord with current recommendations and practice at the time of publication. However, in view of ongoing research, changes in government regulations, and the constant flow of information relating to drug therapy and drug reactions, the reader is urged to check the package insert for each drug for any change in indications and dosage and for added warnings and precautions. This is particularly important when the recommended agent is a new and/or infrequently employed drug.

Printed in Switzerland on acid-free paper by
Thür AG Offsetdruck, Pratteln

Contents Vol. 57, 1992